thefacts

Lupus

SECOND EDITION

also available in the facts series

Eating disorders: the**facts**
FIFTH EDITION
Abraham

Sexually transmitted infections:
the**facts**
SECOND EDITION
Barlow

Thyroid disease: the**facts**
FOURTH EDITION
Vanderpump and Tunbridge

Living with a long-term illness:
the**facts**
Campling

Prenatal tests: the**facts**
DeCrespigny

Obsessive-compulsive disorder:
the**facts**
THIRD EDITION
De Silva

The pill and other forms of
hormonal contraception: the**facts**
SIXTH EDITION
Guillebaud

Myotonic dystrophy: the**facts**
Harper

Ankylosing spondylitis: the**facts**
Khan

Prostate cancer: the**facts**
Mason

Multiple sclerosis: the**facts**
FOURTH EDITION
Matthews

Essential tremor: the**facts**
Plumb

Panic disorder: the**facts**
SECOND EDITION
Rachman

Tourette syndrome: the**facts**
Robertson

Adhd: the**facts**
Selikowitz

Dyslexia and other learning
difficulties: the**facts**
SECOND EDITION
Selikowitz

Schizophrenia: the**facts**
SECOND EDITION
Tsuang

Depression: the**facts**
Wassermann

Polycystic ovary syndrome:
the**facts**
Elsheikh and Murphy

Autism and Asperger syndrome:
the**facts**
Baron-Cohen

Motor neuron disease: the**facts**
Talbot and Marsden

Muscular Dystrophy: the**facts**
THIRD EDITION
Emery

Stroke: the**facts**
Lindley

Osteoarthritis: the**facts**
Arden, Arden, and Hunter

Cosmetic surgery: the**facts**
Waterhouse

thefacts

Lupus
SECOND EDITION

DAVID ISENBERG
Academic Director and Professor of Rheumatology,
Centre for Rheumatology, Department of Medicine,
University College London, UK

SUSAN MANZI
Professor of Medicine and Epidemiology, and
Co-Director of Lupus Centre of Excellence,
University of Pittsburgh, USA

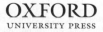
OXFORD
UNIVERSITY PRESS

OXFORD
UNIVERSITY PRESS

Great Clarendon Street, Oxford OX2 6DP

Oxford University Press is a department of the University of Oxford.
It furthers the University's objective of excellence in research, scholarship,
and education by publishing worldwide in

Oxford New York

Auckland Cape Town Dar es Salaam Hong Kong Karachi
Kuala Lumpur Madrid Melbourne Mexico City Nairobi
New Delhi Shanghai Taipei Toronto

With offices in

Argentina Austria Brazil Chile Czech Republic France Greece
Guatemala Hungary Italy Japan Poland Portugal Singapore
South Korea Switzerland Thailand Turkey Ukraine Vietnam

Oxford is a registered trade mark of Oxford University Press
in the UK and in certain other countries

Published in the United States
by Oxford University Press Inc., New York

British Library Cataloguing in Publication Data

Data available

Library of Congress Cataloguing in Publication Data

Data available

ISBN 978-0-19-921387-0 (Pbk.)

10 9 8 7 6 5 4 3 2 1

Typeset in Plantin
by Cepha Imaging Pvt. Ltd., Bangalore, India
Printed in Great Britain
on acid-free paper by
Ashford Colour Press, Gosport, Hampshire

While every effort has been to ensure that the contents of this book are as complete, accurate
and up-to-date as possible at the date of writing, Oxford University Press is not able to give
any guarantee or assurance that such is the case. Readers are urged to take appropriately
qualified medical advice in all cases. The information in this book is intended to be useful to
the general reader, but should not be used as a means of self-diagnosis or for the prescription of
medication. The authors and the publishers do not accept responsibility or legal liability for any
errors in the text or for the misuse or misapplication of material in this book.

Contents

Preface

Systemic lupus erythematosus is a remarkable disease which causes a bewildering variety of symptoms and signs. It may be hard to diagnose, it may be hard to treat, and it can certainly be very difficult to live with. This book is intended to try and help patients, and their relatives and carers, understand more about the origins of the disease, the types of problems that it can cause, and the best ways to try and help patients with different combinations of problems. It also offers hope for the future. We describe the rapid advances in our knowledge of the factors which conspire to cause the disease and how that knowledge is being applied to provide more targeted treatments. We believe that this knowledge will radically alter the way lupus is managed over the next decade. We would both like to thank our family and friends, who have been so supportive during the writing of this book, and in particular, our patients who have inspired it.

David Isenberg
Susan Manzi

Preface

1

What is systemic lupus erythematosus?

⊃ Key points

◆ Systemic lupus erythematosus, though first 'named' in 1851, has existed long before that.

◆ It involves the internal organs, as well as the skin.

◆ It is usually classified or diagnosed on the basis of criteria established by the American College of Rheumatology.

◆ As well as 'classical' clinical features, e.g. photosensitive skin rash, it is also linked to characteristic blood-test abnormalities (e.g. anti-dsDNA antibodies).

The word lupus comes from the Latin meaning wolf and, although rather fanciful, the red and occasionally very unpleasant rashes that may occur on the faces of patients with lupus were said to be reminiscent of a wolf devouring the flesh. Opinions differ as to how long the term has been used, but one suggestion proposes that a monk, Herbernus of Tours, was the first to use it approximately a thousand years ago. Initially, the term seems to have been used in a rather random way but in the last five hundred years it has largely been reserved for skin rashes affecting the face.

The first really clear-cut description of 'discoid' (literally in the round shape of a disc) lupus was that of Laurent Biott in Paris in 1833 (see Table 1.1) and it was his compatriot Pierre Cazenave who first coined the term lupus erythematosus in 1851. For some time thereafter, confusion persisted with the use of the term lupus vulgaris, which is actually a skin rash due to tuberculosis.

Table 1.1 The history of lupus

460–370 BC	Herpes esthiomentoas of Hippocrates. Probably a synonym for SLE – according to Lusitanus (AD 1510–68).
AD 916	Herbernus of Tours in his 'Miracles of St Martin' used the term lupus in a description of the healing of Eraclius.
1230–1611	Rogerius (*c.*1230), Paracelsus (1493–1541), Manardi (*c.*1500), Sennert (1611) all credited with mentioning lupus in their writings.
1845	Hebra first likened the facial rash to a butterfly shape.
1851	Cazenave used the term 'lupus érythémateux', distinguishing it from three other types of lupus.
1872	Kaposi recognizes lupus as a systemic disease.
1904	Jadassohn in Vienna published a 125-page review clearly distinguishing discoid (skin only) and systemic lupus.
1924	Libman and Sacks described an endocarditis now recognized as a form of SLE.
1935	Baehr, Klemperer, and Shirfrin reported structural changes in the glomerulus of lupus patients.
1941	Klemperer, Pollack, and Baehr coined the term 'diffuse connective tissue disorder'.
1948	Discovery of the LE cell test by Hargreaves, Richmond, and Marks.
1949	Thorn and colleagues used cortisone therapy.
1951	Page employed quinacrine (mepacrine), an antimalarial drug, to control lupus with dermal lesions.
1954	Dustan, Taylor, Corcoran, and Page observed that hydralazine could induce LE cells: probably the first report of drug-induced lupus.
1957–58	Friou and colleagues described anti-nuclear antibodies in SLE sera.
1959	Bielschowsky, Helyer, and Howie derived the NZB mouse, the first mouse model of lupus.
1969	Koffler and colleagues correlated immunofluorescent staining patterns of the glomeruli with degree of proteinuria.
1971	American Rheumatism Association published criteria for classification of SLE (revised in 1982 and in 1997).
1976	The first suggestion of Urowitz and colleagues of a link between SLE and atherosclerosis.

(continued)

Table 1.1 The history of lupus (*continued*)

1980–83	Schwartz, Stollar, and colleagues dissected the spectrum of autoantibody-producing cells in both autoimmune mice and humans with SLE.
1980–90	Physicians at the National Institutes of Health, including Klippel, Plotz, and Steinberg, demonstrated the use of combinations of prednisolone and intravenous cyclophosphamide given as boluses for the treatment of severe, especially renal, disease. Hughes, Harris, and colleague identified the important clinical associations of anti-phospholipid antibodies.
1987–93	Combined international efforts undertaken to compare and validate disease activity indices, e.g. BILAG, SLAM, SLEDAI.
1996	Systemic Lupus International Collaborating Clinics (SLICC) agree a validated damage index for SLE.
2000	The first use of a biological agent (rituximab) in the treatment of a lupus patient at University College London.

It was an English physician, Hutchison, in 1873 who first drew attention to the photosensitive nature of the lupus rash. By the early twentieth century, lupus was clearly distinguished as a disease in its own right, occurring in two major forms of discoid, in which only the skin is involved, and systemic, in which the internal organs as well as the skin are affected. The original link between skin and internal-organ disease was made in Vienna in 1872 by Moritz Kaposi.

 Fact

The immune system consists of an army of white blood cells and other cells found in the bloodstream and the body's tissues. Its principal function is to protect the body against invading pathogens, such as viruses and bacteria.

 Fact

Moritz Kaposi is the same Kaposi after whom a form of skin cancer, once rare but now more frequently seen in association with patients who have AIDS, was named.

This historical description does not, however, define the nature of the disease that we now recognize. Systemic lupus erythematosus (SLE) is the consequence of inflammation resulting from an attack by the immune system on the patient's own body, including, ironically, against the immune system itself! There is a simple analogy that helps to explain this. Under normal circumstances whenever we eat, breathe or drink, millions of these pathogens enter our body and, rather like a radar system, the immune system is able to 'scan' and spot these invaders, distinguish them as foreign, i.e. not part of the body, surround and destroy them. The ability to distinguish the body's own tissues (i.e. self), from these invaders (i.e. non-self), is critical to the body's survival. By analogy, during the two Gulf Wars, the American troops at night, on several occasions, shot and killed some of their own forces because in the darkness the troops could not easily distinguish their side ('self') from the enemy ('non-self'). The popular press dubbed this phenomenon 'friendly fire'. This is a good way to look at autoimmune (self-destructive) diseases in general. If the autoimmune attack is directed against the pancreas, the consequence is diabetes; if the attack is directed against parts of the nervous system, the result is multiple sclerosis, and if it is against the adrenal gland, Addison's disease results (Fig. 1.1). The attack against the body's own immune system that occurs in SLE, results in a wide variety of clinical problems ranging from rashes to convulsions, from arthritis to mouth ulcers. No organ or system within the body is entirely safe, although some, notably the skin and joints, are much more frequently affected than others such as the liver or eye.

The vast majority of patients who develop lupus are women (around 90%) and most do so after the onset of periods and before the menopause (thus between 15 and 50 years). However, children and those over 50 may, less frequently, also develop the disease. In these categories, the ratio of females to males is lower – approximately 4:1. The numbers of patients in different ethnic groups also varies. A study in England reported around 40 cases in 100 000 of the Caucasian population; close to 100 per 100 000 in the Asian population (from India, Pakistan and Bangladesh) and just over 200 per 100 000 in the Black population. The figures for Chinese and Hispanic populations are around that of the UK Asian group. Many 'lupus doctors' believe that the disease is more severe in the Black and Chinese populations.

The American College of Rheumatology have produced a set of classification criteria, which are set out in Table 1.2. In order to make a diagnosis of lupus, it is generally accepted that four of these classification criteria should be present. The four (or more) features do not have to be present simultaneously. For example, a patient aged 19 may present with joint pain and swelling (arthritis), have a low white-cell count and a positive antinuclear antibody

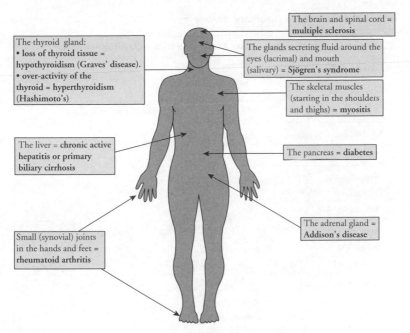

Figure 1.1 Some examples of autoimmune disease – 'sites of attack'.

test (all features suggestive of lupus), but the formal diagnosis must await the development of a fourth feature, say crops of mouth ulcers, which might not appear for another year.

The frequency with which the different clinical features listed as classification criteria, and other commonly observed problems, varies between ethnic groups. For example, white lupus patients are more likely to be sensitive to the light (photosensitive) and thus to develop lupus rashes on a hot summer's day, whereas Black lupus patients have a greater risk of developing kidney involvement.

These criteria also include a number of possible blood-test abnormalities. These include some relatively simple problems, such as a reduction in the number of total white blood cells (leucopenia) and, in particular, a fall in the number of lymphocytes (lymphopenia). In addition, some antibodies (a type of protein described in more detail in Chapter 4), generally known as autoantibodies as they attack the body's own tissues, are key features of SLE.

Table 1.2 Autoimmune rheumatic disease

Criteria of the American Rheumatism Association for the Classification of SLE
1. Malar rash.
2. Discoid rash.
3. Photosensitivity.
4. Oral ulcers.
5. Arthritis.
6. Serositis. Pleuritis. Pericarditis.
7. Renal disorder. Proteinuria >0.5 g/24 h or 3+, persistently. Cellular casts.
8. Neurological disorder. Seizures. Psychosis (having excluded other causes, e.g. drugs).
9. Haemolytic disorder. Haemolytic anaemia. Leucopenia or <4.0 × 10^9/l on two or more occasions. Lymphopenia or <1.5 × 10^9/l on two or more occasions. Thrombocytopenia <100 × 10^9/l.
10. Immunological disorders. Positive LE cell. Raised anti-native DNA antibody binding. Anti-Sm antibody. False-positive serological test for syphilis, present for at least six months.
11. Antinuclear antibody in raised titre.

'. . . a person shall be said to have SLE if four or more of the 11 criteria are present, serially or simultaneously, during any interval of observation.'

Antinuclear antibodies are present in virtually all patients with SLE, although they may be found in the blood of patients with a variety of other diseases, as well as some healthy individuals. More specific for SLE are anti-double-stranded (ds) DNA antibodies and antibodies to a structure known as the Smith antigen, the anti-Sm antibodies. Antiphospholipid antibodies are another criterion and are also commonly present in patients with SLE. However, they too are found in other conditions especially the primary antiphospholipid antibody syndrome (which is characterized by a combination of recurrent spontaneous abortion and a tendency to blood clots).

 Fact

The Smith antigen is a complex combination of RNA and other material derived from the nucleus of cells.

In the next few chapters of this book we will look in more detail at these clinical features and blood test abnormalities identifying those seen early in the disease and will contrast them to others which appear to be late complications.

2

Lupus – what are its early symptoms and signs?

> **Key points**
>
> ◆ Lupus, even in its early stages, can be a chameleon and present in different ways.
>
> ◆ Photosensitive rashes, arthritis, loss of appetite, swollen lymph glands, and pleurisy are common early features.
>
> ◆ The physician needs to think of the possible diagnosis of lupus – and then do the right blood tests to clinch the diagnosis.

As Chapter 1 has emphasized, patients with lupus may, in the course of their 'disease career', develop a wide variety of symptoms and signs. Few patients experience the full range of these problems and, although there are some 'classical presentations' (see below and Fig. 2.1), lupus may, in its early phases, be as bewildering to the physician as it is to the patient.

What then are the early clinical features of lupus and what should family practitioners in particular be looking out for?

The more common presenting features

The most obvious 'classical' form of lupus are patients who present with the so-called 'butterfly rash' (see Fig. 2.1). The rash is named after its shape,

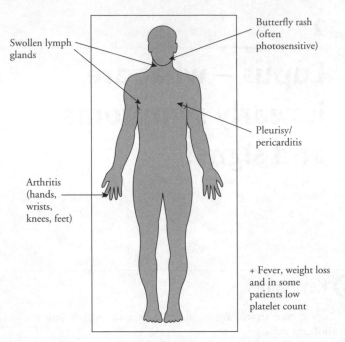

Swollen lymph glands

Butterfly rash (often photosensitive)

Pleurisy/ pericarditis

Arthritis (hands, wrists, knees, feet)

+ Fever, weight loss and in some patients low platelet count

Figure 2.1 Common early clinical features of lupus

since it often involves much of the cheeks with a narrow bridge across the nose, i.e. in the shape of a butterfly. It needs to be distinguished though from other facial skin rashes, notably a condition called rosacea, which is not serious and often responds to antibiotics. The butterfly rash, and other types of rashes, seen in lupus patients are frequently, though not always, exacerbated by sunlight (ultraviolet radiation). The term 'photosensitivity' is used to describe this phenomenon. This history or variations of it are very common. The reason why ultraviolet radiation seems to be linked to lupus are much better understood and Chapter 9 will deal with this important topic.

 Patient's perspective

A young male patient who presented to one of us some years ago described the onset of his lupus:

'I had been invited to take part in a charity boat race on the River Thames, just north of London. It was a very hot day and the boat I was rowing

> in had no protection against the sun, I had no hat and had forgotten to bring any sunscreen with me. My face felt very warm and by the evening the butterfly rash had already developed. I went to see my family doctor the next day and he diagnosed my lupus on the spot.'

The butterfly rash may be accompanied by other distinct 'disc like'/discoid rashes in areas that are also exposed to the sun; for example, over the neck, upper chest, and arms. Ultraviolet radiation does not, however, appear to be the full story, since on occasion patients may present during the winter months with these sorts of rashes and the rashes may extend into areas that were covered by clothing. Nevertheless, any rash largely confined to a sunlight-exposed area must always raise the possibility of lupus as its cause.

Inflammation of the joints often starting with simple aching on movement is another very common feature in early lupus. Joint aching, or arthralgia, usually occurs in the small joints of the hands and sometimes the feet, there afterwards extending to the larger joints, such as the wrists, elbows, and knees. If not recognized, it may go on to develop into real swelling of the affected joints, when the term arthritis is used.

 Fact

The -'itis' at the end of a word, from the Greek, actually means inflammation.

Since the majority of patients with rheumatoid arthritis (a disease roughly 10 times more common than lupus), are also women, it is not surprising that many patients who actually have lupus are initially diagnosed as having rheumatoid arthritis. Although many of the drugs used to treat these two conditions are the same, including corticosteroids, methotrexate, and plaquenil, other drugs such, as gold and to a lesser extent sulphasalazine, have traditionally been reserved for patients with rheumatoid arthritis. Since the outcome of the two diseases is usually very different (rheumatoid affects the internal organs far less frequently, for example) it is important to make the correct diagnosis before inappropriate treatment is given. On clinical grounds alone it may be very difficult to distinguish the early arthritis of rheumatoid and lupus in a young woman, and blood tests and X-rays are invariably required to help make the distinction.

Inflammation of the tissues around the lungs (pleurisy) or heart (pericarditis) are also recognized early features of lupus. These problems typically give rise to pain in the chest (especially at the end of taking a deep breath in) or shortness of breath.

A group of features commonly found early in the course of lupus, and often occurring together, include:

- fatigue;

- fever;

- swollen lymph glands (lymphadenopathy);

- loss of appetite (anorexia); and

- sickness (nausea).

even though they are not listed among the 'official' classification criteria. They may, however, be very troublesome for the patient and, if they are presenting features, may lead physicians 'up the wrong path'. Patients who present with lymphadenopathy and fever, for example, are often extensively investigated for the possibility of a lymph-gland cancer such as lymphoma, also known as Hodgkin's disease, and major infections, notably tuberculosis, before the possibility of an autoimmune condition like lupus is seriously considered. As in much of medicine, context is an essential consideration. Thus, a young, white woman presenting with lymphadenopathy, fever, and joint pains should immediately arouse the suspicion that the underlying diagnosis is lupus (even if, on clinical grounds alone, one cannot make this diagnosis confidently), whereas a young man recently arrived from, say, Bangladesh with a similar history is far more likely to have tuberculosis.

Loss of appetite, which may be linked to weight loss, with or without nausea, may also mislead the physician to think of cancer or chronic infection before considering lupus. In some patients, loss of weight is often linked to flares of lupus. Nausea, if persistent, may result in a host of tests of the gastrointestinal tract, including endoscopy (in which a fibre-optic tube, inserted through the mouth into the oesophagus and stomach, enables the inside of these structures to be visualized).

Precisely how these presenting symptoms are investigated and managed depends upon the healthcare system; these differ significantly in different countries. In the UK, the vast majority of patients presenting with the sort of features described above will go to see their family physicians. In other countries, however, patients tend to go either to the emergency room (casualty) or to a particular specialist. It cannot be emphasized too strongly that the possibility of lupus should be considered in a wide range of clinical presentations among women during the childbearing years. Once thought of it is easy to test for (see Chapter 4) but the initial diagnostic thought is essential.

A distinct subset of patients with lupus present the consequence of low platelet counts.

 Fact

Platelet cells are found in the blood and are responsible for efficient clotting.

If levels of platelets are low, it is likely that easy bruising will result. While somewhat unsightly, bruising in the skin is unlikely to have permanent consequences but the danger is real, if a patient with a low platelet count suffers a fall and knocks their head, since bleeding inside the skull may have serious, and potentially permanent, consequences. Thus any patient presenting for the first time with easy bruising needs to have their platelet count tested very quickly. Only about 5% of patients with lupus present with a major clotting abnormality due to low platelets, but it remains a very important form of presentation. A linked condition, known as idiopathic thrombocytopenia purpura (meaning a low platelet count of uncertain origin), is a relatively common condition and about 15% of these patients go on to get lupus in due course. Unfortunately, there is no way of knowing at the time these patients present, who is going to be among the unlucky 15%!

Other less common presenting features

As the next chapter will emphasize, involvement of the central nervous system is both common in patients with lupus and highly diverse; anything from 'migraine to madness' may be a feature of the disease affecting the central nervous system. However, involvement of this system, at least in a major form, is relatively uncommon. We have seen patients with lupus present with epileptic fits (seizures) and major psychotic episodes (described in more detail in Chapter 3). However, fewer than 5% of patients present in this way and other more typical features of lupus are usually also present. Psychiatric institutions are thus not filled with undiagnosed patients with lupus.

Other even less common presenting features of lupus that we have observed include:

◆ pancarditis (meaning inflammation in each of the main types of tissue in the heart);

- inflammation of the pancreas (pancreatitis); and

- severe vomiting.

We have noticed in our groups of lupus patients that some young men and black women with lupus have a tendency to present with quite severe kidney inflammation (nephritis).

3

Lupus – the chameleon – the clinical features of the disease

Key points

- Lupus is truly a chameleon-like disease and can affect virtually any organ or system in the body.

- Involvement of the skin, joints, lungs, and kidneys are particularly common.

- Involvement of the central nervous system is particularly diverse – anything from 'migraine to madness' can occur (though the latter is very rare).

- Other common, linked conditions include Sjögren's syndrome and anti-phospholipid antibody syndrome.

As already mentioned in Chapter 2, lupus may present with the 'so-called' butterfly rash and the name itself derives from the Latin word meaning wolf, but the animal with which lupus may best be compared is surely the chameleon. Some years ago a young PhD student sat in a lupus clinic with one of us and asked the question, 'Is lupus ever misdiagnosed as another disease'. We asked the first five patients that morning if this had been the case – all five had been misdiagnosed!

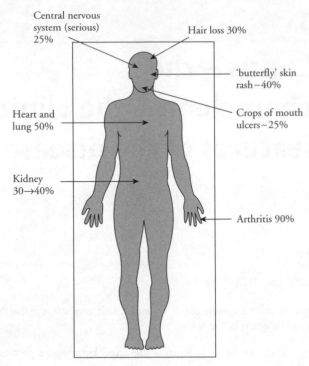

Figure 3.1 Approximate frequency of lupus clinical features.

The problem is that lupus may affect literally any organ or system within the body and must therefore be considered as a possible diagnosis in a wide variety of clinical conditions. In Fig. 3.1, the approximate frequency of clinical features in the different organs and systems is indicated. In this chapter we will consider, in turn, how lupus affects each of these organs and systems, whilst emphasizing that many lupus patients will avoid the majority of these problems during their 'lupus career'.

The skin

The butterfly rash involving the cheeks with a 'bridge' across the nose is the best known of lupus rashes, and perhaps as many as one-third of lupus patients develop this in the course of their disease. The skin typically is red, a little raised, and occasionally blisters. The ridge of skin between the lower edge of the sides of the nostrils and the cheeks (the naso-labial fold) is often relatively spared.

However, the skin, especially fair skin, in patients with lupus is very susceptible to the triggering of a rash following exposure to sunlight (ultraviolet radiation). As a consequence, besides the face, the upper chest, forearms, and hands are also often affected. In very severe cases, large amounts of skin involving a substantial part of the body surface area can be involved – well beyond the area to which ultraviolet radiation normally has access. The sensitivity to ultraviolet radiation is such, however, that lupus patients do run a risk when going on beach holidays or to other hot places in search of a tan. Even driving a car with the window open, allowing access of the sunlight to an arm resting on the open window-frame, can lead to a lupus rash.

In a 'technical sense' there are different varieties of lupus rash with subtle differences in the precise components of the skin tissue that are involved and in the exact causes, but in the main they appear to be the consequence of inflammation of small blood vessels, a process known as vasculitis. This process is integral to the disease itself, the effects simply being more visible on the skin than in the inner organs.

Linked to skin involvement is loss of hair, known medically as alopecia. This may take the form of a generally mild, diffuse type of hair loss (the patient simply notices more hair in the sink after washing and shampooing) or, in less than 10% of patients, there is a severe form of hair loss, which on very rare occasions may involve virtually the whole of the head. For a woman, in particular, severe alopecia is psychologically a disastrous occurrence. Even with the availability of some excellent modern wigs to disguise the problem, it remains one of the hardest aspects of lupus for a patient to deal with day to day. Unfortunately the treatment of alopecia is often unsatisfactory and in severe cases the problem can become permanent.

General features

As described in Chapter 2, patients with lupus may present with fever, weight loss, swollen lymph glands, and even a feeling of sickness and vomiting. These features are easily confused with a wide variety of other conditions, notably forms of cancer of the lymphatic system. These features are not confined to the initial presentation of lupus but may occur as part of a flare at any time. However, even more common than these problems is fatigue.

The importance of fatigue was highlighted to us when at the UCH London lupus clinic a few years ago we carried out a simple survey asking 100 patients to tell us which was the most concerning aspect of their disease. In our naïvety we had assumed it would be fear of death, fear of kidney failure, even fear of a permanent rash–when in fact the feature that concerned the majority of our patients the most was fatigue. And this was not the sort of fatigue associated with 'a good night out,' but a more profound problem. Patients would often tell us that in spite of a good night's sleep, they woke up feeling so exhausted that it was a struggle to take their children to school or they needed to have an additional sleep most afternoons. It certainly made enjoying a social life at night very difficult because they needed to get to bed early.

We are encouraged to believe that fatigue is not a 'mere' psychological problem because the experience of treating patients with rheumatoid arthritis with one of the new biological agents provides us with a telling comparison. These patients are also greatly troubled by fatigue and it is striking that using a TNF alpha-blocking drug, for example, not only eases the pain and swelling of the joints but increases the energy levels of our patients. As we move into the era of biological therapy for our patients with lupus (see Chapters 5 and 10), it will be intriguing to determine whether their fatigue can also be significantly improved in a way that conventional immunosuppression has failed to achieve.

Fever associated with lupus may be very significant (temperatures can exceed 39°C) and it is important to exclude an infectious disease as the cause. Where fevers occur later in lupus, a particular conundrum is that the use of drugs, widely used in patients with lupus, to suppress the immune system (e.g. azathioprine, methotrexate, cyclophosphamide) predisposes patients to infectious diseases. Thus the distinction between a fever due to the disease itself and an infection secondary to immunosuppressive treatment can, on occasions, be very difficult. A blood test known as the C reactive protein (CRP for short) can, though not always, be helpful in resolving this dilemma. The CRP level is usually normal when fever is due solely to lupus disease activity, but high in the presence of an infection. The distinction is not absolute, however, and in some patients with active arthritis or inflammation of the tissues around the heart and lungs, the CRP level may be increased.

Weight loss associated with lupus may also occur at different times throughout the disease course and may be highly significant (exceeding 5% of body weight in a single month). One patient under our care presented with an acute flare on four occasions in approximately 10 years. On each occasion, the flare was associated with a significant degree of weight loss, so that just by looking at the weight-chart it was possible to predict, even before the patient entered the room, what her clinical condition was going to be!

Swollen lymph glands are a common feature of many viral conditions – even an ordinary, common cold is often associated with swelling of the glands beneath the jaw, for example. Swollen glands are also associated with more serious conditions including cancers of the lymphatic system, such as Hodgkin's lymphoma. However, in the majority of patients in whom the cause of the lymph-gland swelling is not sinister, the swollen glands subside back to normal within 4 – 6 weeks. Any patient with swollen lymph glands that persist for more than 6 weeks, needs to be investigated and those investigations may well include a biopsy of the gland.

Swollen lymph glands are thus a common feature of acute flares of lupus, and when biopsies of these glands have been taken, they tend to show mild, inflammatory changes (also known as reactive changes) only. There is no sign of any cancer of the lymphatic tissues. In the main, the swelling of the glands will settle once the flare of the disease is treated with corticosteroids or other immunosuppressive drugs.

Other well-recognized features of flares in patients with lupus, include:

◆ loss of appetite;

◆ feelings of sickness; and even

◆ vomiting.

Whilst perhaps not as common as the other symptoms described above, they can cause diagnostic confusion and may result in patients being investigated with procedures such as abdominal ultrasound, endoscopy, barium swallow, or barium-meal examination just to be sure that there is no underlying problem in the gastrointestinal system.

Central nervous system

The ability of lupus to cause diagnostic confusion is nowhere better illustrated than in the central nervous system. As shown in Chapter 1, the American College of Rheumatology lists just two central nervous system features of lupus as part of the classification criteria:

◆ psychosis – a condition in which patients become very disturbed claiming to hear voices or see visions, which influence their behaviour; a feeling of paranoia, 'people are against me', often accompanies these problems; and

◆ seizures (fits).

In contrast, a working party established by the American College acknowledged that up to 19 different neurological conditions may occur in patients with lupus. This longer list is shown in Table 3.1. Clearly psychosis and seizures are amongst the most troubling of these neurological features.

Fortunately major psychosis in patients with lupus is uncommon, involving probably less than 5% of lupus patients overall, but when it occurs, it is frightening – both to the patient and their caregivers.

Table 3.1 The possible neurological features of systemic lupus erythematosus – proposed by the American College of Rheumatology

Central nervous system
    *Aseptic meningitis
    Cerebrovascular disease
    *Demyelinating syndrome
    Headache (including migraine)
    Movement disorder (chorea)
    *Myelopathy
    Seizure disorders
    *Acute confusional state
    Cognitive dysfunction
    Psychosis

Peripheral nervous system
    *Acute inflammatory demyelinating syndrome (Guillain – Barré syndrome)
    *Autonomic disorder
    *Mononeuropathy
    *Myasthenic gravis
    *Neuropathy, cranial
    *Plexopathy
    Polyneuropathy

*Uncommon <5%.

 Case study

A graphic example was a patient under our care. This highly intelligent woman with a PhD in biochemistry reported quite candidly that she heard threatening voices advising her to kill herself and kill her children.

As she put it:

'The voices seemed very real and seemed to make sense but there was also a restraining voice saying that this was not such a good idea.'

It should be pointed out that this restraining voice is what is lacking in patients with schizophrenia.

The psychosis of lupus also takes other forms. Paranoid delusions, in which patients appear to believe things that clearly do not make sense, and episodes of manic (overactive) behaviour are also well-recorded.

 Case study

As an example, one of the very first patients seen by one of us was a young woman (who subsequently did extremely well), who hardly seemed to sleep, spent much of the day singing at the top of her voice and, given half a chance, would throw glasses of water over approaching staff with the mistaken belief that they were trying to poison her. A combination of steroids and drugs to control the psychosis gradually brought this terrible condition under control, but it did take several months.

There are many different sorts of seizures (fits) of which the *grand mal* seizure is perhaps the best known. As well as losing consciousness, usually for a minute or two, the body shakes quite violently and patients may bite their tongue or pass water without realizing. Probably fewer than 5% of lupus patients actually present with seizures of this type but over the course of a lupus lifetime, probably three to four times as many patients will have at least one such seizure.

Another commonly recognized form of seizure, known as *petit mal*, takes the form of 'minor absences'. In essence, the patient seems to look a little blank and loses 'connection' with what is going on around them, but this state usually lasts for less than a minute.

There are many other forms of epilepsy between these two varieties, depending largely upon which precise part of the brain is 'triggered' during an attack. For example, when the temporal lobe of the brain is involved, the patient will often describe an intense feeling of a familiar smell or sound, or a sense of having been in a similar situation before (*déjà vu*) prior to the loss of consciousness.

The cause of these attacks seems to relate to an irritable part of the brain being triggered, either by the disease itself, some severe form of stress associated with the disease, or possibly other complicating factors. For example, patients with lupus who develop infectious diseases with a high fever may also, on occasion, develop a short-lived or transient form of epilepsy.

A much smaller number of patients with lupus may develop a condition known as peripheral neuropathy. There are two forms of this:

◆ The sensory form of peripheral neuropathy results in the hands and feet becoming numb. There may also be a feeling of pins and needles and the problem may extend up to the forearm and part of the way up the legs.

◆ In contrast, a motor neuropathy causes weakness of the hands and feet, which may lead to great difficulty in performing activities of daily living and make walking and running very difficult.

Lupus patients may suffer partial or complete 'strokes' or cerebrovascular accidents (CVA). These result in the inability to move an arm or a leg or to speak – or all three. There are several possible causes, including high blood pressure which, if left untreated, can cause a bleed in the brain or severe 'furring up' of the arteries in the brain (atherosclerosis) restricting the blood flow and eventually causing the complete cessation of blood flow in blood vessels, which is called a blood clot. High levels of cholesterol in the blood and the presence of antiphospholipid antibodies may contribute to the development of atherosclerosis.

Another serious, but fortunately rare, complication of lupus, also associated with the presence of antiphospholipid antibodies, is a condition known as transverse myelitis. This condition causes inflammation of the spinal cord at a variable level and, because 'nerve signals' run from the brain down the spinal cord and then out to the muscles and blood vessels via the peripheral nerves, the consequence of transverse myelitis is to cause major neurological problems below the level of the inflammation. The degree of disability depends entirely upon the level at which the spinal cord is affected.

 Case study

As an example, seen by one of us, an Egyptian doctor, 3 years after the onset of her lupus, complained of numbness in a band around the middle of her waist. She was unable to stand and could not feel the light touch from a piece of cotton wool below this level. She also became incontinent of both urine and her bowels. Tragically her condition of transverse myelitis was not recognized soon enough. Treatment was given too slowly and she remained in a wheelchair until she died about three years later. Fortunately, this is a rare condition occurring in just three patients among the first 400 looked after at University College London over a 25-year period.

By far the commonest neurological problem recorded by patients with lupus is headache, especially migraine headache. There is some debate in the literature as to whether or not this is truly a feature of lupus or just a common problem that happens to occur in patients who also have lupus. Similarly, anxiety and depression are commonly found amongst patients with lupus, but whether this is really due to the disease or simply the natural manifestation of a reasonable concern about having a potentially serious condition, is also not entirely resolved. Corticosteroids have a somewhat euphoric effect (a feeling of intense happiness) in some patients or cause irritability in others and this too may add to the difficulties in terms of neurological assessment.

Musculoskeletal involvement

Over 90% of patients with lupus develop problems with their joints and/or muscles. The word 'arthritis' implies true inflammation with swelling of the joints, and swollen hands and feet are often reported by lupus patients. 'Arthralgia', in contrast, simply means pain of the joints but without any accompanying swelling. This problem is even more common in lupus patients and may also be accompanied by aching in the muscles or myalgia. Pain and/or swelling in the joints and muscles may lead to great difficulty with carrying out the ordinary activities of daily living, ranging from making a cup of tea to peeling potatoes or laying the table. Although the joint pains of lupus tend to be less persistent than those of rheumatoid arthritis, the combination of the severe fatigue of lupus and intermittent, occasionally constant, joint and muscle pain often combine to make patients depressed and irritable.

Occasionally the swelling of the joints, especially the knees, is sufficient to warrant the aspiration (removal) of fluid from within the joint. This process is often accompanied by the injecting of local steroid into the joint, which is usually a highly effective form of treatment.

True muscle inflammation, myositis, which is associated with weakness of the muscles around the shoulders and hips, is uncommon. Around 4% of the lupus patients seen at University College London have also had myositis

Because rheumatoid arthritis and lupus are both more common in women, and because both commonly begin before the age of 50, many lupus patients are initially misdiagnosed with rheumatoid arthritis. A key distinguishing feature is that the vast majority of patients with rheumatoid arthritis, especially if untreated for more than a few months, develop small holes, known as erosions in their bones. This problem is far less commonly seen in lupus patients (<5%). A little confusingly, both conditions may be associated with the presence in their blood of an antinuclear antibody (see Chapter 4) and a positive rheumatoid-factor test. However, whereas close to 100% of lupus patients have a positive antinuclear antibody, usually at a very high level, a positive antinuclear antibody test is seen in only 25% of rheumatoid arthritis patients. In contrast, whereas 70% or more of patients with rheumatoid arthritis have a rheumatoid-factor test, amongst lupus patients the figure is 20–25%. Additional tests may be needed to help resolve the problem, thus antibodies to double-stranded DNA are present in 60–70% of patients with lupus but very rarely found in patients with rheumatoid arthritis. In contrast, a test for the anti-CCP (cyclic citrullinated protein) antibody is virtually never seen, except in patients with rheumatoid arthritis. Nevertheless, on occasions it may be difficult to be sure at the start of the disease which condition patients really have, although this usually becomes clear within the first few months of follow-up.

Cardiovascular-respiratory disease

Involvement of the lungs and, to a slightly lesser extent, the heart, are commonly recognized problems in patients with lupus. Both organs are surrounded by thin layers of tissue that may easily become inflamed in the course of a lupus flare. The pleural tissues around the lungs, when inflamed, cause a distinct pain, usually at the end of taking a deep breath in (inspiration). In more troublesome disease, fluid may collect between these tissue layers around the lung giving rise to a condition known as a pleural effusion, which can cause severe shortness of breath. In a similar way, the lining or pericardial tissues around the heart can cause central chest pain, which often varies according to the position of the body and can usually be distinguished from the chest pain of angina (see below). The tissues around the heart may also become a site for a collection of fluid known as a pericardial effusion. This may interfere with the normal beating of the heart and can also cause shortness of breath.

As well as the lining layers around these organs, the lung and heart tissues themselves may, on occasions, be involved in the disease process. Lung involvement in the heart takes a variety of forms, but in essence inflammation within the lung tissues can lead to permanent damage with the laying down of fibrous tissue causing, for example, a condition known as fibrosing alveolitis. Alternatively there may be inflammation in the lung tissues themselves – a condition known as pneumonitis. The clinical feature most commonly associated with both of these problems is increasing shortness of breath. Internal lung disease is much more difficult to treat successfully than the inflammation of the lining tissues around the lung.

In a similar way, involvement of the heart tissues, both the heart muscle and the valves of the heart, which help to direct the flow of blood, can also have serious consequences.

> ## ❗ Fact
>
> The heart is divided into two upper chambers, the right and left atria, and two lower chambers, the right and left ventricles. Blood returning to the heart through a large vein, the vena cava, flows directly into the right atrium. From the right atrium the blood passes an important valve, the tricuspid valve, into the right ventricle. From there the blood flows to the lungs (in order to remove carbon dioxide and to collect oxygen) before flowing back into the left atrium past the mitral valve into the left ventricle and from there the heart pumps blood out into the aorta and via this major blood vessel all around the rest of the body.

In the 1920s, two American doctors Libman and Sacks first reported small growths, also known as vegetations on the heart valves of patients with lupus. Although uncommon, when this problem does occur, the flow of blood through the heart may be interfered with leading ultimately to heart failure.

Even more importantly, it has been confirmed by several studies in the past 30 years that lupus patients are far more prone to the development of atherosclerosis. This is a complex problem affecting blood vessels but can be compared with the way that water-pipes may become 'clogged up' and eventually blocked over the years. The important 'pipes' in this case are the blood vessels in the heart muscle itself. When this blood supply is interfered with, small portions of the heart muscle tissue may die causing a heart attack, also known as a myocardial infarct. As reported from the lupus clinic in Pittsburgh, lupus patients between the ages of 35 and 45 are 50 times more likely to have a heart attack than aged-matched controls. An important research question still unresolved is why patients with lupus have this increased risk. The conventional risk factors for the development of atherosclerosis include:

- smoking;

- family history of heart attacks or strokes;

- high blood pressure;

- high cholesterol levels; and

- diabetes.

Apart perhaps from high blood pressure levels (usually secondary to kidney disease), patients with lupus do not appear to have increased conventional risk factors. However, it is vital that any identifiable risk factors, such as high levels of cholesterol or blood pressure, that can be corrected, should be corrected. Smoking needs to be strongly discouraged.

Thus there are likely to be factors particular to lupus patients that are responsible for this problem. One possibility is that the presence of the high levels of antiphospholipid antibodies may well be associated with the increased risk of atherosclerosis, and is thus a very important blood test (biomarker) to check in all patients with lupus. Another possibility relates to an enzyme called paraoxonase, which normally 'holds in check' the tendency of blood-vessel walls to become lined with what are known as 'foam cells', which help to form part of the 'fur' on blood vessel walls. It has been shown that patients with lupus have a lowered level of this enzyme. The full explanation for the increased risk of atherosclerosis is not yet elucidated, though it is likely to be multi-factorial.

The kidneys

 Fact

The kidneys are essential organs in the body as they organize the filtering and removal of the waste products from the blood into the urine, which passes through two tubes, known as the ureters, into the bladder and from there to the exterior via the urethra tube.

Approximately one-third of patients with systemic lupus have major inflammation in their kidneys and if this is not treated can lead to kidney failure which, before the introduction of dialysis and kidney transplantation, led, in turn, to death. Manifestations of kidney disease are invariably identified by simple urine tests and other investigations, rather than by problems that the patient is aware of – at least until very substantial damage has been done. The dipstick test, for example, identifies the presence of excessive amounts of protein and blood in the urine, problems that, unless the blood loss is very heavy, the patient is often unaware of. Likewise high blood pressure, often linked to impaired kidney functioning, is frequently a 'silent problem' and has to be formally measured.

Kidney involvement in patients with lupus takes several forms. A kidney biopsy can reveal minimal changes only or inflammatory changes in a confined area (focal) of the glomeruli.

Fact

Glomeruli are the portions of the kidney where waste fluids pass out of the blood system into the tubular system that will become the ureter.

More generalized involvement of the glomeruli (diffuse proliferative change) may occur and this is the most serious form. Other forms are recognized, including the 'so-called' membranous nephritis, and some patients actually present with profound scarring in the kidney, at which point little can be done to alter the likely failure of the kidneys to function.

Kidney disease in lupus is thus very important and can, if not treated adequately, become very serious. As a routine in our clinics we check the urine of our lupus patients on every occasion. Likewise, regular measurement of the blood pressure is essential; the successful management of kidney disease is critically dependent upon the successful control of blood pressure. In many patients with lupus, kidney disease becomes obvious within the first 1–3 years. Occasionally patients who have had the disease for a decade or more, without any evident involvement in the kidneys, quite suddenly develop significant amounts of protein in the urine and are found to have active kidney disease. The widespread use of steroids, immunosuppressive drugs, and antihypertensive drugs has helped to bring about a reduction in end-stage kidney failure.

In later chapters we will describe in more detail kidney dialysis and kidney transplantation, but we need to emphasize here that these two types of treatment have revolutionized the outcome for patients with lupus as a whole. These procedures became more widely available from the late 1970s onwards and have undoubtedly contributed to the far greater longevity of patients with SLE now compared with 50 years ago.

The blood system

Many patients with lupus suffer from low levels of haemoglobin (a key protein found inside red cells that carries oxygen around the body), white blood cells, and platelets. These problems can have a profound effect upon the general health of the patient. A low level of haemoglobin in patients with lupus, which contributes to the sense of fatigue, can have a variety of causes including:

◆ what is known as the 'anaemia of chronic disease';

◆ the presence of antibodies against some component of red blood cells (this can be diagnosed by an investigation known as the Coombs' test); or

♦ the side-effects of drugs used to treat patients with lupus; for example, non-steroidal anti-inflammatory drugs, such as voltarol (Diclofenac) and naprosyn (Naproxen), can irritate the lining of the stomach and cause blood loss.

The more powerful immunosuppressive drugs, such as cyclophosphamide and azathioprine, may on rare occasions damage the bone marrow (from the where the blood cells actually come from) and also lead to anaemia.

The white blood cells are essential to the normal defence of the body against bacteria, viruses, and fungi. Around 40% of lupus patients have a low level of total white cells but around 80% have low levels of a particular type of white cell known as the lymphocyte cell. Lupus patients are thus less well-protected from infectious organisms and, unfortunately, the use of many drugs that suppress the immune system, while very helpful in controlling flares of lupus, can also add to this increased risk of an infection.

Platelets are the cells involved in producing a blood clot following a cut. Without sufficient numbers of these cells, there is a tendency to bleed – on occasions quite severely. Low levels of platelets (a condition known as thrombocytopenia) can occur as an isolated event some years in advance of the development of other features of lupus (as discussed in Chapter 2). On occasions, low levels may be found as a part of an acute disease flare – often in association with the presence of antibodies to the platelet surface membrane. Some patients, notably those with high levels of antiphospholipid antibodies, may have a chronically low level of platelets, which can be difficult to treat. The presence of antiphospholipid antibodies is somewhat paradoxical here since their presence may be associated with an increased risk of clotting notably when total platelet numbers are not affected.

The liver and spleen

The liver is the largest organ in the body but is relatively uncommonly involved in systemic lupus. The liver produces a variety of enzymes and measuring these by a blood test can be used as a simple way to check on whether the liver is actually 'under attack'. An ultrasound examination is another simple way of assessing the liver. Although liver-function tests are relatively often increased in patients with lupus, detailed studies have suggested that probably fewer than 10% of lupus patients actually have significant disease of the liver. Autoimmune hepatitis and autoimmune biliary cirrhosis are occasionally seen in patients with lupus and these conditions may require immunosuppressive therapy. The majority of liver-enzyme abnormalities, however, are probably due to complications of some of the drugs used to treat the disease. This is particularly true when patients are being treated with methotrexate or non-steroidal anti-inflammatory drugs.

The spleen, which is to be found close to the left-hand side of the stomach beneath the rib cage, is also rarely involved in patients with lupus. It may be a little swollen in perhaps as many as 5% – 10% of lupus patients but this gives relatively few symptoms and it is unusual for a physician to be able to palpate a swollen spleen in patients with lupus, although an ultrasound examination may show it to be a little enlarged.

The eye

The commonest form of eye involvement in lupus is the cataract – a form of opacity in the optic lens, partially interfering with vision; this is a complication of steroid therapy rather than an effect of the disease itself. Lupus disease truly affecting the eye is rare. Occasionally, the retinal blood vessels (the retina is at the back of the eyeball) may become inflamed (retinal vasculitis) and this may cause a serious impairment in vision, which can be hard to treat successfully.

Sjögren's syndrome (named after a Swedish ophthalmologist) affects around 10% of all patients with lupus. This disease, caused by the inflammation and eventual destruction of the fluid-producing glands around the eyes and mouth, results in their becoming profoundly dry. The eyes become red, itchy, and irritable, and the patient finds bright light uncomfortable. Patients waking at night may find it difficult to open their eyelids. Infections of the eyes may become a problem and every effort must be made to keep the eyes as moist as possible. This is usually achieved by the regular use of artificial tear drops (preferably preservative-free), though a minor operation is sometimes undertaken to help keep the eyes from becoming dry.

The gastrointestinal tract

The gastrointestinal tract involves the mouth to the anus. Although Crohn's disease may involve any part of this system, lupus patients rarely have involvement beyond the stomach; mouth ulcers are by far the commonest feature. Although mouth ulcers are quite common in the general population, around a quarter of all lupus patients have troublesome, recurrent crops of quite painful ulcers, usually found on the roof of the mouth, and on the tongue, which may be hard to eradicate.

The effects of Sjögren's syndrome (see above) on the mouth can be very irritating. The persistent dryness of the mouth makes gum disease (infection and even shrinkage of the tissues) a particular problem. Unless a major effort is made to minimize the use of drinks with high-sugar content, increased tooth decay and the need for more dental fillings are inevitable. As with the eyes, every effort must be made to keep the mouth as moist as possible. Many patients find it helpful to carry a bottle of water with them at all times and to take frequent sips. Drugs such as pilocarpine may help some patients and various artificial saliva replacements solutions are available.

Some lupus patients suffer a form of overlap syndrome with a form of scleroderma and this may be associated with malfunction of the valve that guides the contents of the oesophagus in to the stomach. As a consequence, the acid contents of the stomach may 'spill over' into the lower oesophagus, whose lining cell layer is not 'built' to deal with them. This difficulty, known as reflux oesophagitis, may result in central chest pain and require the regular use of antacid preparations.

Many lupus patients use non-steroidal anti-inflammatory drugs and these may irritate the lining of the stomach leading both to stomach cramps and pain–and, less frequently (as above), to major stomach bleeds.

Involvement of the small and large intestines is rare in lupus patients but occasionally vasculitis, affecting the blood vessels that supply these tissues, may occur. This is a potentially dangerous situation causing severe abdominal pain and may require surgery to remove the affected tissues.

4

Tests for diagnosing and managing lupus

> **➲ Key points**
>
> - A variety of tests are needed to help make the diagnosis of SLE, notably blood tests. Some, for example, the antinuclear antibody test, whilst commonly found (95%), are not specific; others like anti-dsDNA (50–60%) and anti-Sm (10–30%) are less common but are virtually specific.
>
> - A wide variety of tests from imaging (e.g. chest X-rays, CT scans) to electrical tests (e.g. EMG) are needed to assess the effect of lupus on the different organs and systems.
>
> - Certain blood and urine tests will be performed at virtually every out-patient/office visit to help monitor both effect of the disease and to ensure that the drugs prescribed are not causing any side-effects.

Lupus has been described as a mysterious disease. It has earned this title in part because it may be difficult to diagnose. Unfortunately, there is no one test developed specifically to detect lupus. Because lupus can present differently in every patient, and many signs and symptoms of lupus can mimic other diseases, patients may go years before a proper diagnosis is made. Patients with lupus are like snowflakes, with no two exactly alike. This chapter will review the most common tests that are carried out when a diagnosis of lupus is suspected. We will also review the blood tests that are commonly ordered in patients with established lupus for monitoring disease activity.

We will discuss these tests in two major categories:

1. We will review the tests obtained to determine whether a patient has specific organ involvement, such as kidney disease, inflammation of the lining of the heart or lungs, or blood-cell abnormalities.

2. We will then discuss the blood tests that measure autoimmunity. These latter tests are not routinely performed in patients without auto-immune diseases.

Tests to evaluate organ-system involvement

Although, the tests described are commonly used to diagnose lupus and to determine which organ or systems of the body are being affected by lupus, they are also frequently done throughout the course of the disease to monitor lupus activity in each of these organ systems. It would not be uncommon for your doctor to obtain blood and urine tests at all of your routine visits. Many of these tests will detect abnormalities before there are obvious physical signs or symptoms. This is particularly true of blood cell abnormalities and kidney disease.

The musculoskeletal system

This is the most common organ system involved in lupus. The most common musculoskeletal problem is joint pain (arthralgia) with or without swelling, tenderness, morning stiffness, and warmth (arthritis). Arthritis is most easily detected during physical examination, but sometimes an X-ray or bone scan of the joints may help make the diagnosis.

The skin

Skin is the second most commonly affected organ in lupus. Some lupus rashes can look like other skin diseases. When there is uncertainty about whether the rash is due to lupus, a small skin biopsy is obtained. It is such a small biopsy that it has been termed a 'punch' biopsy, since it is a quick and, generally, painless procedure done in the office or out-patient clinic. There are common findings suggestive of lupus that can be found on the biopsy, including special patterns of inflammatory cells deposited in certain layers of the skin.

Blood cells

Blood cell abnormalities are very common in patients with lupus. When lupus is suspected patients are evaluated for evidence of anaemia or low red-cell blood counts, low white cell blood counts and low platelet counts. This often requires obtaining a complete blood count.

Kidney

Several tests can be done to determine if a patient has kidney disease. The first and simplest test is a urinalysis, which involves examining a urine specimen for the presence of red blood cells, white blood cells, and structures called cellular casts. Analysis of the urine can most easily be undertaken using a 'dipstick'. This is a small plastic stick on which small amounts of chemicals have been fixed that are able to detect protein, blood, and glucose, amongst other things. Casts in the urine reflect kidney disease and can be seen under the microscope. Often the urinalysis provides the earliest detection tool for kidney disease. In addition, your doctor will probably check your blood for creatinine. This is a product produced by the muscles that is removed by the kidney. If someone has loss of kidney function due to lupus, increases in the blood levels of creatinine can be measured. If protein is detected on a simple urinalysis, you may be asked to collect a 24-hour urine sample for measurement of the total amount of protein that is eliminated in the kidney over a full day. (It is also possible to achieve a reasonably accurate estimate of protein loss on a single or 'spot' sample.) The 24-hour urine sample also provides a way of measuring kidney function.

If any of these tests are abnormal, and your doctor suspects that lupus has affected your kidney, you may be asked to undergo a kidney biopsy to determine if there is inflammation in the kidney itself. The kidney biopsy can also guide your doctor as to the type of treatment that may be most appropriate. Often, before a biopsy is performed, you may have an ultrasound or sound wave test of the kidneys to guide the physician who will be doing the biopsy.

Liver

Less frequently, lupus can involve the liver. Often, doctors will check your blood for evidence of inflammation or elevation in certain proteins released from the liver. Rarely, an ultrasound scan of the abdomen, to look at the size of the liver, may be undertaken.

Heart and lungs

If patients present with chest pain or shortness of breath, suggesting inflammation around the heart and lungs, your doctor may send you for an echocardiogram or sound-wave test of your heart, to look for fluid around the lining of the heart.

You may also have a chest X-ray or CT-scan of your lungs to look for fluid around the lining of the lungs. Lung function can also be tested using a piece of equipment known as a spirometer, which requires the patient to exhale (blow out) as hard as possible into a tube that connects to the machine. It can measure the total lung capacity and the ability of the lung to exchange gases (oxygen is generally taken into the body on inspiration and carbon dioxide on expiration) efficiently.

Brain and spinal cord

Some patients will present with lupus involving the brain. In rare cases, lupus patients can have transverse myelitis (inflammation of the spinal cord). This condition may cause weakness or loss of sensation in the legs. Sometimes it is in a stocking distribution or the area that would be covered by a pair of socks or stockings. An equivalent loss of sensation can occur in the arms – in a so-called glove distribution. Often the tests obtained to detect abnormalities in the central nervous system (brain and spinal cord) include a CT-scan or magnetic resonance imaging (MRI) of the brain or spinal cord along with a spinal tap. Spinal fluid can be evaluated for evidence of inflammation or activation of the immune system, suggesting that lupus may be targeting the brain. If a lupus patient has a convulsion or seizure, an electroencephalogram (EEG) is usually ordered. This test can detect seizure activity in the brain that may not be obvious at the time of the examination.

Sometimes the nerves and muscles of the extremities (arms and legs) can be affected by lupus. This may result in numbness and tingling in the hands and feet (similar to what was described with central nervous symptom problems above) or muscle weakness. Blood tests to measure a protein (CPK) released from inflamed muscles and an electromyelogram (EMG), a test to confirm that the muscles or nerves are abnormal, are helpful in making the diagnosis. The EMG test identifies muscle abnormalities by inserting a thin 'recording' needle electrode via the skin into different muscles. Abnormalities of the nerves are identified by positioning skin electrodes over different parts of a peripheral nerve and seeing how long an electrical discharge takes to pass from one to the other. If abnormalities on the EMG are detected, you may be asked to undergo a biopsy of the nerve or muscle to confirm that the problem is due to inflammation from your lupus.

Measurements of autoimmunity

The presence of certain antibodies to self (autoantibodies) can help in the diagnosis of lupus. The most commonly obtained autoantibody is an anti-nuclear antibody (ANA). A screening test for ANA is routine when a diagnosis of lupus is suspected. An ANA is present in about 95% of patients with lupus. Unfortunately, ANAs are not specific to lupus and can be seen in many other autoimmune and infectious conditions, and in approximately 10–15% of healthy women. If the ANA is positive, there are other autoantibody tests that can be obtained (see Fig. 4.1), which are more specific for lupus. One of those antibodies is to double-stranded DNA (anti-dsDNA). This test is highly specific for lupus and is not found in patients with other rheumatic diseases. About 50–60% of lupus patients will have this antibody present. This means that there are many patients with lupus who do not make this antibody. The presence of antibodies to dsDNA is associated with lupus kidney disease.

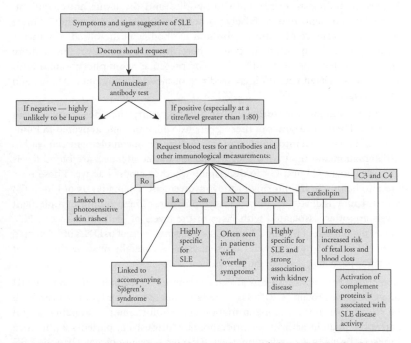

Figure 4.1 Autoantibody testing pathway in patients with SLE. NB Ro/La/Sm/RNP are known collectively as the 'extractible nuclear antigens'.

Other specific autoantibodies include antibodies to Smith (anti-Sm). This is an antibody that is rarely found in patients with other rheumatic diseases but is present in only about 30% of patients with lupus. Some patients with lupus may have antibodies to ribonuclear protein (RNP) or a rheumatoid factor (RF). In many cases these antibodies are seen in patients with features of other autoimmune conditions along with their lupus, including scleroderma, polymyositis or Sjögren's.

Antibodies to Ro (SSA) and La (SSB) can also be detected in about 30% of patients with lupus. These antibodies are often seen in patients with skin rashes brought on after sun exposure and in mothers who have had babies with what is known as 'neonatal lupus'. These antibodies are frequently checked prior to pregnancy, since mothers have to be monitored carefully for neonatal lupus. More about this condition is discussed in Chapter 7.

Some lupus patients have antibodies that react to phospholipids. Phospholipids are found in many tissues of the body. These antibodies have been termed antiphospholipid antibodies. There are several types of antiphospholipid antibodies, including anticardiolipin antibodies and the lupus anticoagulant. Some lupus patients may be falsely positive for a blood test for syphilis. This is due to the presence of antiphospholipid antibodies in the blood of patients with lupus. It is important in cases where this test is positive, that a more specific test for syphilis be obtained. The presence of antiphospholipid antibodies is associated with an increased risk of blood clotting, fetal deaths, and miscarriages.

Another common measurement of autoimmunity includes complement proteins. There are a series of these proteins, which become activated in lupus and can break down into tiny fragments. Activation of complement can lead to inflammation and tissue damage. Physicians frequently measure blood levels of complement C3 and C4 to determine whether lupus is active. These tests are also helpful in monitoring kidney involvement. Falling levels of blood C3 and C4 may indicate an impending lupus flare. These falling complement levels are often associated with rises in the levels of antibodies to dsDNA. When the pattern of falling C3 and C4 and rising levels of dsDNA are detected in the blood of a patient with lupus, physicians carefully observe the patient for flares particularly involving the kidney.

Sometimes your physician may check an erythrocyte sedimentation rate (ESR) or a C-reactive protein (CRP). These tests are not specific for lupus but can both be elevated when there is inflammation present, for example, in patients with active rheumatoid arthritis or pneumonia. Curiously, in patients with active lupus, in the absence of infection, the CRP often remains normal when the ESR is raised. Inflammation can be present during lupus flares or active infections. It is important to distinguish the reason for the elevation in these markers.

Summary

There are many blood tests, including those routinely obtained to determine which organ systems of the body are being affected by lupus, as well as blood tests evaluating the autoimmune response. In addition to these blood tests, biopsies and other imaging tools can be useful for both diagnosis of lupus and monitoring of disease activity. There has been great interest recently in developing new blood tests or biomarkers, including:

- genetic factors;

- complement protein activation products, which deposit on circulating blood cells; and

- other specific proteins that may be elevated in lupus patients when the disease is active.

We are hopeful that, with the development of better biomarkers for lupus, we will be able to more accurately:

- diagnosis lupus;

- identify individuals at risk for getting lupus;

- identify those patients who may benefit from specific treatments; or

- identify those who may be at greatest risk for a having a lupus flare.

5

Treatment

> ## ⮕ Key points
>
> ◆ In the past 50 years a number of drugs have been used to treat patients with SLE, ranging from antimalarials to immunosuppressives, which do offer significant benefits.
>
> ◆ These drugs do not help every patient and it is important to find the right combination for the individual patient, at any given point in the course of their disease.
>
> ◆ There is constant need to monitor the benefits of these drugs against the side-effects they can cause.
>
> ◆ Although the treatment of lupus is vastly improved compared with 50 years ago, there is an obvious need to develop new drugs better targeted at the molecules that actually cause the disease.

People with lupus are living longer and healthier lives due to major advancements in treatment over the past 50 years. There still remains room for improvement. Fortunately there are novel new treatments on the horizon that more precisely target the molecules we now believe contribute directly to the cause of lupus. The goal of these new therapies is to reduce inflammation and favourably alter the autoimmune response, while limiting side-effects. In general, treatment should be customized for each patient depending on the organ system involved and the severity of the disease. In this chapter we will review the commonly used medications for lupus and describe the rationale for some of the newer therapies being developed. We will discuss approaches for the management of lupus that do not involve drugs in another chapter.

Non-steroidal anti-inflammatory drugs (NSAIDS)

Non-steroidal anti-inflammatory drugs (NSAIDs) are effective in pain relief and are widely used in lupus for problems including arthritis, inflammation of the lining of the heart and lungs, headaches and muscle pain (see Table 5.1).

Table 5.1 Drug therapy in systemic lupus

	NSAID	Anti-malarial	Cortico-steroids	Immunosuppressive agents
Fever	+	−	+	−
Pleurisy or pericarditis	+	−	+	−
Joint pain	+	+	+	−
Joint pain with swelling and warmth	+	+	+	+
Muscle pain	+	+	+	−
Muscle weakness with inflammation in the muscle tissue	−	−	+	+
Rash	−	+	+	−
Inflammation of the lung tissue (pneumonitis)	−	−	+	+
Vasculitis	−	−	+	+
CNS disease*	−	−	+	+
Kidney	−	−	+	+
Haemolytic anaemia	−	−	+	+
Low platelet count	−	−	+	+

* This depends on the type of brain involvement. Many strokes require a blood thinner and/or aspirin.
Note: +, usually beneficial; −, not generally beneficial.

Fact

On an historical note, aspirin was the first NSAID to be developed. It became widely available from 1899 having been synthesized a year or so earlier by a technician, Felix Hoffman, who worked for the Bayer company in Germany. Remarkably, in the same month that he synthesized aspirin, he also synthesized heroin!

The effectiveness of these drugs varies among patients and can change in the same patient over time. These medications can reduce inflammation and control pain. Possible side-effects include:

◆ stomach upset;

◆ impairment of kidney function;

◆ impairment of liver function.

Patients on these agents should be carefully monitored for these potential side-effects. In general however, NSAIDs are relatively safe and widely used (see Table 5.2 for common side-effects).

In patients with kidney impairment, NSAIDs should be avoided, since the inhibition of the enzyme cyclooxygenase (COX) by NSAIDs can further impair the blood flow to the kidneys. There is a special type of NSAID, called the selective COX-2 inhibitor, which reduces the gastrointestinal (GI) side-effects, namely peptic ulcers and bleeding. However, due to the increased risk of blood clotting and cardiovascular events (heart attacks) in selective COX-2 users, these agents should generally be avoided in patients with known coronary heart disease or those at high risk for having a blood clot. Since many patients with lupus are considered to be at high risk for heart disease and blood clots, we generally avoid using these agents unless absolutely necessary. In those cases, we add a daily aspirin. Only one selective COX-2 inhibitor (celecoxib) remains on the current market.

In contrast to the increased clotting risk with the selective COX-2 inhibitors, there are antiplatelet effects with the non-selective COX inhibitors (e.g. naproxen, ibuprofen, etc.). Non-selective COX inhibitors should be discontinued prior to surgery to avoid bleeding complications and should be used sparingly in the setting of blood-thinners. NSAIDs should not be used during the last 3 months of pregnancy due to potential harm to the baby's heart (see Table 5.2 for the use of common drugs during pregnancy).

Table 5.2 Potential side-effects of drugs used in systemic lupus erythematosus

Drug	Adverse reactions	Pregnancy
NSAIDs	GI* bleed, inflammation of the liver and kidneys, high blood pressure, headache, non-infectious (aseptic) meningitis.	Discontinue in third trimester (last 3 months).
Corticosteroids	High blood pressure, abnormal cholesterol levels, elevated blood glucose, cataracts, loss of blood supply to the joint bones (avascular necrosis), osteoporosis.	Safe use the lowest dose.
Antimalarials (hydroxychloroquine, chloroquine, quinacrine)	Pigment changes on the retina, GI complaints, rash, muscle pain, headache; haemolytic anaemia in patients with G6PD deficiency.†	Safe.
Dapsone	Haemolytic anaemia in patients with G6PD deficiency.	Discontinue 4 weeks before delivery.
Azathioprine	Bone marrow suppression, inflammation of the liver, blood cell cancers.	Safe.
Methotrexate	Mouth sores, bone marrow suppression, inflammation of the liver, cirrhosis, inflammation of the lungs.	Teratogenic.‡
Cyclophosphamide	Bone marrow suppression, irritation and bleeding in the bladder, cancer, infertility.	Teratogenic.
Mycophenylate mofetil	Bone marrow suppression, GI complaints (diarrhoea).	Limited information, should avoid.
Cyclosporine	Bone marrow suppression, thickening of the gumline, inflammation of the liver, kidney impairment, abnormal cholesterol.	Generally safe, but may consider switching to azathioprine.

* GI, gastrointestinal.

† G6PD glucose-6-phosphate dehydrogenase.

This enzyme can be measured in a blood sample prior to starting anti-malarials or dapsone.

‡ Teratogenic – causing birth defects.

Corticosteroids (prednisone, prednisolone, medrol)

- Corticosteroids (prednisone, prednisolone, medrol) are effective in the treatment of various inflammatory rheumatic diseases and can provide immediate relief of many manifestations of lupus. These agents can be used as a cream or lotion on the skin (topically), by mouth (orally), as an injection into the skin, muscle or joint, or by vein (intravenously). Generally, the intravenous administration is reserved for severe manifestations of lupus. Corticosteroids are quite effective in managing:

- skin rashes;

- arthritis;

- inflammation of the lining of the heart and lungs (pericarditis and pleurisy);

as well as more serious manifestations, including:

- kidney involvement (nephritis);

- inflammation of the lung tissue itself (pneumonitis);

- haematological (blood cell) abnormalities; and

- central nervous system (brain and nerve) involvement.

There are differences in the doses of prednisolone given to patients with lupus to treat the various clinical features. In broad terms, patients with arthritis, pleuritis (inflammation of the tissues lining the lungs) and pericarditis (inflammation of the tissues around the heart) will often be started on doses of 20–30 mg. In contrast, patients with severe nephritis, very low platelet counts or very low haemoglobins (due to active lupus) will often be treated with at least twice as high a dose. Many patients will require a 'steroid maintenance dose of 5–10 mg for many months after the acute problem has been brought under control.

Although corticosteroids are extremely effective, they have numerous side-effects that include:

- weight gain

- increase in blood pressure and blood sugar levels;

- increase in risk of infection

- bone thinning;

- bone infarcts (avascular necrosis),

- cataracts; and in some cases

- gastritis; and

- GI bleeding.

The use of corticosteroids alone is less concerning than in combination with NSAIDs, where the frequency of GI bleeding and ulcers goes up significantly For these reasons, physicians should use the least amount of corticosteroids, carefully weighing the risks and benefits.

Antimalarial agents (hydroxychloroquine, chloroquine, quinacrine)

Antimalarial agents are one of the most commonly used drugs to treat lupus. Hydroxychloroquine (HCQ) is the agent most frequently prescribed, followed by chloroquine and quinacrine. The antimalarials generally do not work as quickly as corticosteroids and may take several months to reach full effectiveness. Hydroxychloroquine, introduced in 1955, was found by chance to be effective in treating lupus and rheumatoid arthritis. It is usually dosed at 200 mg/day or 200 mg twice daily. Dosing often depends on the weight of the individual and many side-effects can be avoided if doses remain at, or below, 6.5 mg/kg body weight. Chloroquine is used at 250 mg/day (3.5 mg/kg/day) with effects seen within 3–4 weeks sooner than that of HCQ. Quinacrine, which has a rapid onset of action similar to chloroquine, is usually dosed at 100–200 mg/day (2.5 mg/kg/per day). Combination therapy with HCQ (or chloroquine) and quinacrine is commonly used with success when one agent alone is not effective.

Antimalarial agents are best at treating:

- skin rashes;

- joint pain;

- fatigue;

- other mild manifestations of lupus.

Gastrointestinal (stomach) side-effects are the most common, but are usually temporary and can be reduced by lowering the dose of the antimalarial agent. A very rare but important potential side-effect of the antimalarials is retinal toxicity. Pigment can be deposited on the retina (back of the eye) and can cause changes in vision. The current recommendation is for patients taking antimalarials to have eye examinations before starting the drug and then every 6 – 12 months thereafter.

Another precaution when taking antimalarials is the risk of haemolytic anaemia (red blood cells are destroyed in the circulation) in patients with glucose-6-phosphate dehydrogenase (G6PD) deficiency. G6PD deficiency is more common in the Mediterranean regions, Middle East, Africa, and the Indian subcontinent, and can be easily detected in a simple blood test. Other potential effects from antimalarials include hyper-pigmentation (darkening) of the skin. This most commonly occurs on the front part of the lower legs or shins. Sometimes patients may mistakenly complain of 'bruises' that don't go away. There are other benefits of antimalarial agents beyond control of lupus disease activity.

- ◆ First, hydroxychloroquine has been shown to be safe during pregnancy.

- ◆ In addition it can reduce blood sugar levels and has been helpful in some patients with type II diabetes. Patients should be aware of this sugar-lowering effect, which in some patients may result in light-headedness after taking the medication.

- ◆ Hydroxychloroquine may also reduce lipid levels, and may be mildly protective against clotting events.

Because the antimalarials are generally safe and effective, with added benefits beyond the treatment of lupus, these agents are widely used. An important fact that many patients are not aware of is that cigarette smoking may interfere with the efficacy of antimalarials in treating discoid lupus and other lupus skin rashes. Improvement of skin lesions can occur once patients stop smoking and remain on antimalarial therapy. This is another reason to stop smoking... not that you need any more reasons!

Dapsone

Dapsone is a sulfone antibiotic traditionally used in the treatment of leprosy. Once again, we have fallen upon a drug that is designed to treat one disease, but is very effective in treating certain features of lupus, particularly skin rashes!! Dapsone (100 mg/day) alone or in combination with systemic corticosteroids/antimalarials, is the drug of choice for bullous SLE (blistering skin lesions), as well as for cutaneous vasculitis (inflammation of the small blood vessels in the skin).

Similar to antimalarials, patients with G6PD deficiency are at increased risk of developing haemolytic anaemia while taking dapsone. Although dapsone is not teratogenic, it can increase the risk of blood-cell abnormalities in the foetus and discontinuation of dapsone therapy 1 month before the expected date of delivery is recommended. Breast-feeding by mothers taking dapsone should be cautioned, since this drug is secreted in breast milk and can place the infants at risk of developing haemolytic anaemia.

Immunosuppressive agents

These medications are generally used to allow physicians to reduce the dose of corticosteroids and to provide additional suppression of the autoimmune response in patients with more severe disease. Because these drugs are potent suppressors of the immune system, they may increase a patient's risk for infection. It is important for patients and doctors to be aware of this risk and to evaluate carefully for infections, when appropriate. There has always been a theoretical concern about development of cancer in patients who take potent immuno-suppressive agents. The theory has been that these agents interfere with the immune system's ability to properly guard against the formation and spread of cancerous cells. There is rather convincing evidence that taking oral (by mouth) cyclophosphamide daily for a prolonged period of time can lead to bladder irritation, bleeding, and, in rare situations, bladder cancer. However, the case against the other immunosuppressive agents as inducers of cancer is weak. Recent studies conducted by the Systemic Lupus International Collaborating Clinics (SLICC group) have failed to show any strong association between immunosuppressive agents and cancer risk in thousands of lupus patients from around the world.

We will describe the most commonly used immunosuppressive agents here.

Azathioprine

Azathioprine at doses of 2–2.5 mg/kg/per day is effective in treating moderate to severe disease activity, including kidney disease and other organ-threatening manifestations. One of the advantages of azathioprine is that it can be safe-ly used during pregnancy in women at risk of serious lupus flares. The main side-effect of azathioprine is suppression of the bone marrow, although occasional liver-function abnormalities may be seen. Regular monitoring of blood counts and liver function tests is recommended.

Methotrexate

Methotrexate has been the standard treatment for rheumatoid arthritis for many years. It is also effective in treating many manifestations of systemic lupus. It is particularly helpful in patients with lupus who are suffering from arthritis, skin rashes, and may allow reduction in corticosteroid dosing. Common side-effects of methotrexate include:

- gastrointestinal complaints;

- mouth sores;

- mild hair thinning; and

- inflammation of the liver.

Patients taking methotrexate should be advised against regular alcohol consumption, since a combination of methotrexate and alcohol can further increase the risk of liver damage. A rare but potentially life-threatening lung complication is methotrexate-induced pneumonitis (inflammation of the lung). Discontinuation of methotrexate is warranted when either pneumonia or methotrexate-induced pneumonitis is suspected. The addition of folic acid (B-vitamin) 1–2 mg on a daily basis usually 5–6 days per week, may reduce the occurrence of common side-effects. There is an injectable (shot) form of methotrexate that can be used in patients with severe stomach upset. Methotrexate should NEVER be used during pregnancy, since it has been associated with significant birth defects in babies. It should be discontinued 3–6 months prior to pregnancy.

Cyclophosphamide

Cyclophosphamide is a potent immunosuppressive agent used to treat severe lupus, including:

- kidney and central nervous system disease;

- inflammation of the lung (pneumonitis); and

- systemic vasculitis.

In the 1980s, the National Institutes of Health (NIH) conducted studies as a result of which cyclophosphamide (in high dose given by intravenous, i.e. into the vein, infusion monthly for 6 months then every 3 months for 2 years) became the gold standard for treatment of a severe form of lupus kidney disease. The use of this agent along with corticosteroids reduced the occurrence of kidney failure. Although cyclophosphamide is clearly effective in treating lupus, it has many potential side-effects. Common ones include:

- nausea, which can easily be controlled with the newer anti-nausea medications now available;

- mild hair thinning;

- bone marrow suppression; and

- a small but real risk of bladder irritation, bleeding and in rare cases bladder cancer.

Cyclophosphamide is eliminated from the body by the kidneys and can be toxic to the bladder. For these reasons it is important for patients receiving cyclophosphamide to remain well hydrated to flush the medication from their system more effectively. An unfortunate side-effect of cyclophosphamide can be ovarian failure resulting in infertility. This is most commonly seen in women over 30 who have received higher total doses of cyclophosphamide. In Europe, studies using two weekly infusions of cyclophosphamide at much lower doses have been equally effective at treating lupus kidney disease. Overall, current practice is to use the smallest amount of cyclophosphamide necessary to get the disease under control and then to switch to less toxic medications to maintain the improvement.

Mycophenylate mofetil (MMF)

MMF is an agent now available that appears to be very effective in treating lupus kidney disease and other serious manifestations of lupus. MMF has been used widely to prevent kidney transplant rejection. There have been several encouraging studies showing that MMF is as effective as cyclophosphamide in treating active lupus kidney disease. MMF is generally well-tolerated at the dosing range from 500 to 1500 mg twice daily. Side-effects include gastrointestinal complaints (nausea, bloating, and diarrhoea), and bone marrow suppression. The gastrointestinal reactions can be minimized by gently increasing the dose of MMF. MMF promises to be an excellent alternative to cyclophosphamide for the treatment of kidney disease, particularly in young women where fertility issues are important.

Cyclosporine

Cyclosporine was introduced as a drug to prevent organ-transplant rejection, but like so many of our other drugs it also has a role in the treatment of lupus. Dosages of cyclosporine ranging from 2.5 to 5 mg/kg/per day are generally well-tolerated and may allow reduction of corticosteroid dosage and improvement in lupus disease activity. A recent study showed that cyclosporine was as effective as azathioprine in managing lupus flares. Most side-effects are dose-dependent and reversible. The most serious side-effects include kidney abnormalities and worsening hypertension. Regular monitoring of kidney function and blood pressure are advised. Limited pregnancy data, primarily from transplant patients, showed no increase in adverse outcomes in pregnancy. Cyclosporine can be continued in pregnant patients with SLE if the benefits outweigh the risks. Mothers taking cyclosporine are advised against breast-feeding since cyclosporine passes into breast milk.

Other treatments

Other less commonly used treatments for lupus include intravenous immuno-globulin (IVIG), which is most helpful in treating extremely low platelet counts, which may be associated with serious bleeding.

Plasma exchange or plasmapheresis is rarely used these days, being reserved generally for very specific conditions associated with lupus. This treatment involves removing and filtering the blood of patients with lupus to remove cir-culating autoantibodies. The most common reason for using plasmapheresis in lupus is to treat thrombotic thrombocytopenia purpura, which is a rare con-dition resulting in low platelet counts, kidney problems, fevers, and seizures. Plasmapheresis is sometimes used for life-threatening complications of lupus when conventional therapy has failed.

In severe cases of SLE that do not respond to traditional immunosuppressive therapy, stem-cell transplantation has been used. This procedure involves high doses of intravenous cyclophosphamide followed by infusion of the patients own bone-marrow cells (autologous stem cells). This procedure is designed to 'reset' the immune response by eliminating the current immune cells and starting over with early immune cells from the bone marrow. Autologous stem cell transplantation has shown promise for patients with severe disease, but there is risk for serious complications around the time of the procedure.

Dialysis and kidney transplantation

The availability of dialysis and kidney transplantation has improved survival of patients with SLE. In the not so distant past, lupus patients who had kidney failure died. Now with the availability of dialysis and transplantation, these same patients are living longer. Aside from an increased risk of infection, SLE patients generally do well with dialysis. For those patients who undergo kidney transplan-tation, long-term outcomes are similar to those transplant patients without SLE.

Novel new treatments

This is an exciting time for new drug discovery in lupus. The general principal of the novel new therapies is moving away from 'global' or total suppression of the immune system toward 'targeted' therapies that focus on the immune system abnormalities specific to lupus. This has the potential to improve the effectiveness and lower the side-effects. There are many new agents currently being developed and evaluated in clinical trials (research studies of new drugs). These novel agents can target various steps in the autoimmune process.

B cells

Many of them are directed at B cells, which are specific immune cells responsible for making autoantibodies (antibodies to self) in lupus. One promising new drug is Rituximab, which binds to a receptor on the surface of B cells (CD20) and causes the B cell to die. Rituximab is a monoclonal antibody approved by the Federal Drug Administration (FDA) in the USA for the treatment of non-Hodgkin's lymphoma and rheumatoid arthritis. Many patients with lupus have been treated with Rituximab with promising results. This drug is currently being evaluated in hundreds of patients with lupus in several clinical trials.

LJP 394 is another agent directed at B cells that make antibodies to DNA (a common antibody in patients with lupus). This agent prevents the B cell from making new antibodies. Results of a clinical trial in SLE patients with kidney disease showed that LJP 394 had very few side-effects and in a small group of patients was able to prevent a flare of kidney disease.

B-cell activating factor (BAFF)/B-cell stimulator (BlyS) helps B cells survive. In patients with lupus, this results in persistent formation of autoantibodies. Belimumab is a human BAFF monoclonal antibody that blocks these factors and prevents survival of B cells. Early studies showed that belimumab may reduce disease activity in lupus. Additional clinical trials are underway.

T cells

In order for B cells to make autoantibodies (antibodies to self), they need to communicate with T cells. This communication requires interlocking of molecules on the surfaces of B and T cells. Once this binding occurs, the B cell can continue to 'pump out' autoantibodies. Abatacept is a fusion protein that interrupts the B cell–T cell signalling and thus prevents formation of autoantibodies. This drug has been approved by the FDA for the treatment of rheumatoid arthritis. Multicentre clinical trials are currently under way in SLE.

Cytokine blockade

When B and T cells are stimulated or activated, they help produce substances that cause inflammation and tissue damage. These substances are called cytokines. Some new therapies are designed to block the action of cytokines to directly reduce inflammation and tissue damage. Perfect examples of very effective cytokine inhibitors are the tumour necrosis factor (TNF-α) inhibitors (etanercept, infliximab, and adalimumab). These agents have been extremely successful in treatment of rheumatoid arthritis and psoriatic arthritis. A small open-label study of infliximab in SLE showed significant improvement in patients with severe kidney disease that did not respond to standard treatment. One concern about using these agents in lupus has been the observation that a few patients with rheumatoid arthritis who are on TNF-α inhibitors develop antibodies to DNA (a common antibody seen in lupus). Fortunately, even fewer of them actually develop a lupus-like illness. Clinical trials are needed to determine the safety and efficacy of this therapy in SLE.

Interleukin 10 (IL-10) is a cytokine that may participate in the pathogenesis of SLE. A small open-label study of six SLE patients using a monoclonal antibody against IL-10 showed improvement of skin and joint symptoms. However, all of the patients developed antibodies against the monoclonal antibodies, which were developed in mouse models.

Interleukin 6 (IL-6) is another cytokine that causes inflammation. It also stimulates B cells and T cells. Tocilizumab is a humanized monoclonal antibody against IL-6 receptor (IL-6R) that suppresses IL-6 activity. IL-6 blockade is currently being tested in patients with SLE.

Elevated serum levels of interferon-a are found in patients with SLE and the presence of this inflammatory cytokine is increased when disease activity is high. The observation that people can develop a lupus-like illness on interferon-a therapy for unrelated conditions supports the concept that this cytokine plays an important role in lupus pathogenesis. Decreasing levels of interferon-a may be another promising treatment for SLE.

Summary

Treatment for lupus has come a long way over the past 50 years and has resulted in significant improvement in patient survival and quality of life. We are hopeful that over the next 5–10 years there will more effective and safer treatment options available for patients with lupus. The complexity of lupus and the wide range of severity in different organ systems will likely translate into the need for a variety of treatment options.

6

Treatment that does not involve drugs

> ## ➡ Key points
>
> ◆ There are many important things that patients with lupus can do 'beyond' drugs to help them manage their disease.
>
> ◆ Avoiding direct sunlight, minimizing stress, and a balanced diet are all helpful.
>
> ◆ Do not have 'live viral' vaccines if you are on more than 10 mg prednisolone and/or immunosuppressive drugs.
>
> ◆ Non-adherence in treatment carries health risks.

Many patients ask if there are things that they can do beyond taking medication to manage their lupus. The short answer to this question is yes – many things (see Fig. 6.1). In this chapter we will discuss some of the most common 'non-drug' management tips.

Learn about lupus

Becoming educated about lupus and the treatment for lupus is fundamental to proper management of the disease. Education gives you more control of your condition and allows better communication with your doctor. Your rheumatologist can guide you to the sources that will provide the best educational material. It is important to provide a cautionary note here. Many patients have already begun their own investigation through the vast information highway of the internet. Although there is sound information provided through the internet, there can be many inaccuracies, particularly on websites with no oversight by qualified healthcare professionals. Some of the information can

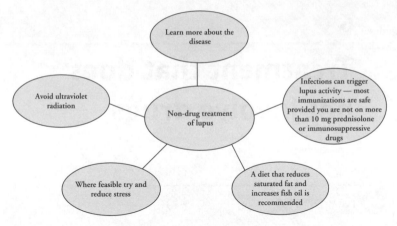

Figure 6.1 Non-drug therapy for SLE.

generate confusion and fear. Even well-intentioned friends and family members may provide erroneous advice regarding lupus and its management. It is critically important that patients establish a trusting relationship with a physician or a healthcare professional, who is knowledgeable about lupus, and to go to them for advice and guidance. Remember that education is power, but only if it is accurate.

Avoid things that can trigger a lupus flare

Ultraviolet light

There are environmental triggers that can cause lupus to flare. One of the most recognized is exposure to ultraviolet light or sunlight. This is called photosensitivity or sensitivity to the light. Exposure to ultraviolet light can result in increased fatigue, skin rashes, joint pain, and even internal organ inflammation in patients with lupus. There is now scientific evidence to explain how sunlight can cause a lupus flare. Ultraviolet light can cause our skin cells to undergo cell death. This is what happens when we get sunburn. When skin cells die, they release proteins that are normally safely tucked away in the cell and hidden from our immune system. When these 'self-proteins' are released from the dying skin cells, they can generate an autoimmune response in patients with lupus, and trigger a lupus flare. It is important for lupus patients to protect themselves from excessive sun exposure. This includes avoiding sunlight during mid-day when the sun is the most intense, using sunscreens and sun blocks and, in some cases, photo-protective clothing and hats. Even driving a car with your arm exposed on an open window can cause trouble.

There are window films and fluorescent light shields available that can also reduce ultraviolet light exposure and minimize the risk of a lupus flare. Patients need to know that certain drugs can increase sensitivity to the sun, including commonly used antibiotics. Extra precautions should be made if taking these medications.

Stress

It is well-known that stress caused by tensions at work, worry about children, marital problems, financial issues or even anxiety about moving into a new home can affect our immune system and possibly increase lupus disease activity. It is unrealistic to think that we can completely eliminate stress from our lives. There is no 'stress-ometer' by which we can easily measure stress and clearly individuals vary greatly in their ability to cope with difficult situations.

There are ways to reduce stress that can be beneficial to everyone, particularly patients with lupus. One of the most effective ways of reducing stress is with physical activity. Exercising may be easier when your lupus is less active and you're feeling better, but gentle range of motion exercises and walking can even be done during a flare. Exercise can not only prevent muscle weakness and improve your cardiovascular health, it has a tremendous affect on reducing stress, anxiety, and even depression. A physical therapist can work with you to set up a reasonable exercise programme that fits your schedule and takes into account any physical limitations. This can often be as easy as designing a walking programme.

Many patients have found that biofeedback, yoga, and even acupuncture, performed by trained professionals, can reduce stress and fatigue. The first step is recognizing that stress can affect your lupus, then it is up to you to choose a programme to reduce stress and improve relaxation that is best for you. Remember that small steps forward, as long as you stick to it, are the most successful. Don't become discouraged, soon you will discover the major benefits of exercise, stress reduction, and relaxation on your health.

An important but often overlooked component of managing lupus is the attention to the psychological affects of the disease. There can be many emotional problems that go hand in hand with having a chronic disease. In some cases, professional counselling may be most helpful. More details regarding living and coping with lupus will be provided in another chapter.

Infections and immunizations

Patients with lupus are more susceptible to infections, both due to the nature of the disease itself or its treatment may trigger a lupus flare. This increased risk of infection is made worse by the medications that we use to suppress the autoimmune response and treat the disease. For these reasons, fevers in lupus patients may be more serious than in those without lupus. Patients are advised to seek medical attention for unexplained fevers and not immediately blame the fevers on lupus flares.

Many patients have questions and concerns regarding the safety of immunizations. In general, patients with lupus tolerate immunizations well without any adverse reactions. There have been a few reports of some patients experiencing a flare in their disease following an immunization, but this association has not been proven. It is true that immunizations may be less effective in patients with lupus, particularly those on high doses of corticosteroids or other immunosuppressive agents. Immunizations with killed vaccine (e.g. influenza, tetanus, pneumococcus) are considered safe. The safety of live vaccines (e.g. polio, mumps, measles, rubella, and yellow fever) in lupus patients on high doses of corticosteroids (more then 10 mg prednisolone per day) and other immunosuppressive drugs has not been confirmed and should be avoided. In addition, lupus patients should avoid close contact for about 2 weeks with any person who has received a live vaccine.

Other management and prevention strategies

Diet, heart, and bone health

We are what we eat; a cliché that is absolutely true. Eating a balanced diet, even when your appetite might not be good, is an important component of the treatment programme. If you have kidney disease related to your lupus, your doctor may recommend a low-salt diet to prevent fluid retention or to control your blood pressure. Sometimes you may be asked to limit your protein intake, depending on the type of kidney disease that you have. Some patients with lupus have high levels of homocysteine, a protein that has been linked to heart disease. Your doctor may ask you to take folic acid, a B vitamin, which can reduce the levels of homocysteine.

In general, all patients with lupus should take a multivitamin, unless there is a specific reason not to. Multivitamins provide your body with the necessary nutrients that it may be missing, particularly during times when your appetite is low and your diet is not optimal. Maintaining a healthy body weight is more important than we previously realized in treating lupus. There is recent evidence that visceral or internal organ fat content can increase inflammation. A study revealed that lupus patients on a strict low-fat diet (saturated fat content less than 25%) along with fish-oil supplementation did better with regard to their lupus than those on a regular diet with olive-oil supplementation. We may soon learn that obesity may also increase the risk of developing inflammatory conditions such as lupus.

Because lupus patients are at a significantly increased risk for heart disease (nearly 8–10-fold higher risk than expected), a diet low in fat and cholesterol is imperative beyond the possible benefits of reducing disease activity. Cardiovascular-disease prevention should be a part of the routine care for patients with lupus. Smoking is a major risk factor for heart attack and stroke, and under no circumstances should patients with lupus use tobacco. If quitting is too difficult to do on you own, ask your doctor about joining a smoking-cessation programme.

People with lupus are at increased risk for osteoporosis or bone thinning. This may be due to the inflammation associated with lupus, which can increase bone loss, as well as the medications used to treat lupus, particularly cortico-steroids. In any case, prevention measures are becoming critically important. This includes calcium and vitamin D supplementation. In some cases, prescription medications called bisphosphonates may be needed.

Adherence to therapy

Even with the development of more effective therapies to treat lupus, many patients are not enjoying the full benefits of these treatment advances. One of the reasons for this may surprise you. It is called 'non-compliance' or 'lack of adherence' to prescribed medications. This means that many patients do not take the medications that their doctors prescribe. Not only do they not take their medications, but they often are embarrassed to admit this to their doctors. The reasons for not taking medications may include unpleasant or embarrass-ing side-effects, difficulty remembering to take the medication, the belief that it will not help, and, in some cases, the cost may be too high. Any of these reasons may be justifiable, but if your doctor does not know, he or she will incorrectly assume that the drug does not work. This may lead to your doctor prescribing more potent and potentially more toxic therapies for something that may have been treated using less. In addition, this may put you at increased risk for a lupus flare, hospitalization, or other bad outcome that could be avoided with proper treatment. In a recent study in London it was reported that 50% of patients whose kidneys failed were non-adherent to their recom-mended medicines.

Missing a dose of your medication here or there is usually not a critical error, but it is in your best interest to discuss these issues with your doctor. There may be solutions that are agreeable to both of you, such as using a weekly pillbox or changing the dosing of your medication to one that you can more easily remember. In some cases, it may be treating the side-effect so that you can continue to take what may be a very effective treatment for your lupus. Ask your doctor to fully explain the benefits of the treatment in a way that will help you to understand the importance of taking your medication. Don't be embarrassed to tell your doctor the truth. Together you can develop a strategy that will give you the best chance of reaching maximum benefit from your medications.

Summary

There are many things that lupus patients can do to gain control of their disease. Becoming educated about lupus, as well as avoiding triggers of lupus flares including sun exposure, stress, and infections, are important management tools. A healthy diet, exercise, and prevention of heart disease and bone loss are equally important in maintaining a healthy lifestyle. Remember, medications will not help you if you are not taking them correctly!! Together, these strategies can have a huge impact on the quality of life of people with lupus.

7

Lupus in special situations (children, elderly onset, drug-induced lupus, and pregnancy)

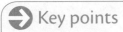 Key points

- Lupus occurring in children causes similar types of clinical features to that found in adults but there are special problems relating to growth and the need to overcome particular problems of poor adherence.

- Lupus occurring in those over 55 is associated with an increased risk of damage.

- The best chance of a good outcome for pregnancy in lupus patients is to ensure that they have been in remission for some time before conceiving.

- Co-managing a pregnancy with a rheumatologist and obstetrician is strongly advised.

Although lupus primarily targets women between the ages of 15 and 45 years, young children and older adults may also develop lupus. Some medications can cause a lupus-like illness. These special situations warrant further discussion.

In addition, this chapter will focus on lupus during pregnancy, which can present unique challenges.

Lupus in children and adolescents

About 20% of all patients who have lupus are diagnosed in childhood. This most often occurs during adolescence, since lupus is rare in children less than 5 years of age. It is interesting that, although most affected patients are female, the female-to-male ratio changes with age. Before puberty, it is three females for every one male diagnosed with lupus; while after puberty, it is closer to nine to one. This observation has prompted interesting research examining the role of hormones on the onset of lupus. Although, lupus in children is basically the same disease as in adults, with similar clinical features, the care of children and adolescents may be very different. Healthcare providers must consider the special needs of these young people and their families, including the psychological and physical changes that are taking place at these ages.

 Fact

The most common presenting symptoms of lupus in children include:

- fever;

- weight loss;

- malaise (general feeling of being unwell); and

- joint pain.

Children often have evidence of arthritis with swollen and tender joints on examination, kidney problems with excess protein and inflammatory cells present in the urine, and mouth ulcers. In addition, haematological or blood-cell-related abnormalities are also frequently present, involving white blood cell, red blood cells, and platelets. If the nervous system is affected, children may complain of headaches or present with more serious abnormalities, including seizures, strokes, or chorea (a type of involuntary movement of the arms and legs). It is not uncommon for adolescents to experience a decline in academic performance or experience social isolation. It is often difficult to distinguish behavioural changes due to lupus from the normal difficulties seen with many teenagers. Sometime during the course of the disease, up to 75% of adolescents will have inflammation of the lining of the heart or lung, which results in chest pain with breathing and shortness of breath.

The diagnosis and treatment of lupus in children is similar to adults in most cases, thus medications such as cyclophosphamide can result in ovarian failure and infertility. If these drugs are needed, minimizing exposure is strongly recommended.

However, children and adolescents present several unique problems related to their growth and development. First, corticosteroids (prednisone, prednisolone, medrol) can have a significant affect on bone growth and result in delayed development and short stature. In addition, the prognosis of lupus in children and adolescents who are diagnosed early and receive proper treatment can be quite good. However, it is critical to recognize that individuals in this age group are often in denial and have a tendency to stop their medications because of a desire to be 'normal' like all of their other friends. The fear of any changes in their physical appearance, such as weight-gain from corticosteroids or hair loss from lupus or its treatment, can be devastating and can result in less compliance. Many of these children also require support from parents, other family members, and teachers. A team approach to management results in much better outcomes in children with lupus.

Lupus in the elderly

Several studies have suggested that the age of an individual when they are diagnosed with lupus is an important factor that can influence how lupus presents and the course of the disease. Some experts believe that when lupus is diagnosed in an older individual the disease may be milder with a better prognosis. 'Older age' in these studies has generally been considered between the ages of 50 and 60 years (this is a highly debatable point from your ageing authors' perspective!). In more recent work conducted by an international group of lupus experts, the notion that late-onset lupus is more benign was challenged. In this study, patients who were diagnosed after the age of 54 were defined as the late-onset group and were compared with patients who were diagnosed at an earlier age. These groups of patients were followed for 5 years to determine the outcomes related to lupus and/or its treatment. The results suggested that there was more evidence of organ damage (meaning a permanent change) in the late-onset group, compared with the younger group, followed over the same 5-year period. It should be pointed out that this 'damage' in the organ systems could be a result of lupus, the treatment for lupus, or, importantly, the natural ageing process.

The late-onset lupus patients were more likely to have:

♦ cataracts;

♦ deforming arthritis;

♦ osteoporosis (bone thinning) with bone fractures;

and cardiovascular manifestations, including:

♦ angina;

♦ heart attack; and

♦ coronary artery bypass surgery.

In general, we now believe that late-onset lupus should not uniformly be judged as more 'benign' than lupus that develops at an earlier age. It is quite possible that lupus accelerates the natural ageing process and may increase the frequency of damage in different organ systems with increasing age.

Drug-induced lupus

Drug-induced lupus is a condition caused by a reaction to certain medications. Men and women at any age can develop the condition. The signs and symptoms of drug-induced lupus are similar to systemic lupus but tend to be a bit milder and go away when the drug is stopped.

Medications most commonly associated with drug-induced lupus are:

♦ anti-seizure medications;

♦ thyroid medications; and

♦ drugs to treat acne.

Lupus and pregnancy

Lupus occurs most commonly in women of childbearing age (15-45 years). Fortunately, women with lupus rarely have problems with fertility and can become pregnant at similar rates to women in the general population. However, pregnancies in lupus women may be associated with complications. The outcomes for mothers with lupus and their children are best when the mothers' lupus is under control with no evidence of disease activity. This makes careful planning of anticipated pregnancies critically important.

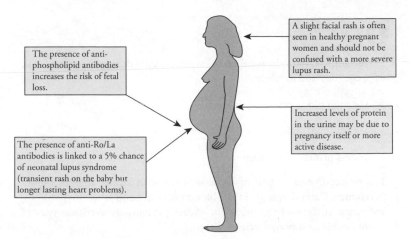

The presence of anti-phospholipid antibodies increases the risk of fetal loss.

A slight facial rash is often seen in healthy pregnant women and should not be confused with a more severe lupus rash.

Increased levels of protein in the urine may be due to pregnancy itself or more active disease.

The presence of anti-Ro/La antibodies is linked to a 5% chance of neonatal lupus syndrome (transient rash on the baby but longer lasting heart problems).

Figure 7.1 SLE – the problems with pregnancy.

What happens to mothers with lupus who are pregnant?

Some experts believe that lupus flares are increased during pregnancy, while others say they are not. Lupus is characterized by periods where the disease is quiet followed by periods with increased activity. This pattern appears to be no different whether the patient is pregnant or not. Having said that, it is critical to point out that the likelihood of having a flare during pregnancy appears to be dependent on how active lupus is at the time a woman becomes pregnant. Most studies suggest that women who have been in remission (no disease activity) for at least 6 months prior to becoming pregnant have a much better chance of not having a flare during their pregnancy. This emphasizes the importance of family planning and avoidance of unexpected pregnancies.

Pregnancy may impose an additional burden on women with a previous history of kidney disease. Pregnancy can place additional stress on the kidneys and can result in worsening of kidney function. It is important for women with kidney disease to have control of their lupus and blood pressure prior to becoming pregnant. While there is some controversy about the effect of pregnancy on disease activity in lupus, there is convincing evidence that pregnancies in lupus women are more likely to be complicated. This includes:

◆ increased rates of pre-term delivery;

◆ blood clots; and

◆ pre-eclampsia.

Fact

Pre-eclampsia, sometimes called toxaemia, occurs during the second-half of pregnancy and involves:

◆ elevated blood pressure;

◆ leg swelling; and

◆ excess protein in the urine.

It may occur in over half of lupus women with kidney disease before pregnancy. Careful monitoring of blood pressures and laboratory studies, including analysis of the urine for excess protein, are a critical part of monitoring lupus pregnancies.

A general rule of thumb is that if the mother remains healthy during the pregnancy, the baby has a much better chance of doing well. Because of this, physicians are more likely to keep lupus mothers on medications to control their disease throughout the pregnancy, including hydroxychloroquine and other immunosuppressive agents that are safe during pregnancy. These decisions must be made on a case-by-case basis, and the risks and benefits of maintaining these medications should be discussed.

What happens to the babies of mothers with lupus during pregnancy?

Fortunately, the frequency of foetal loss appears to be declining. The highest risk still remains in women with:

◆ uncontrolled elevated blood pressure;

◆ lupus kidney disease;

◆ active lupus at the time of pregnancy; and

◆ those with certain antibody markers in their blood, which include elevated levels of anti-DNA antibodies.

Other important antibodies associated with foetal loss include antiphospholipid antibodies (anticardiolipin antibodies and the lupus anticoagulant). These antibodies are associated with sudden miscarriage.

Mothers who have antibodies to Ro/SSA and/or La/SSB are at increased risk of having babies with neonatal lupus. This condition results when antibodies from the mother cross the placenta and interfere with the development of the baby. Fortunately, most cases of neonatal lupus are temporary and result in a mild skin rash in the baby during the first 6 months of life. However, in a small percentage of cases, these antibodies can interfere with development of the heart and can result in heart block. Congenital heart block is a condition that causes abnormalities in how the baby's heart beats. If the heart block is mild, no treatment is needed. In more serious cases, placement of a pacemaker at the time of delivery to help the heart beat at appropriate time intervals may be needed. It is important for all mothers who have antibodies to Ro/SSA or La/SSB to be monitored with foetal echocardiograms (sound wave tests of the foetal heart) after the sixteenth week of pregnancy and through the delivery of the baby. This provides the obstetricians with an opportunity to detect any abnormal heartbeats before the baby is born. The neonatal specialists should also be prepared to examine the baby carefully and use a heart pacemaker, if needed, after delivery.

Although most mothers with lupus will do quite well during pregnancy and deliver healthy babies, it is important to anticipate any potential problems ahead of time so that appropriate treatments can be given. Prior to becoming pregnant, women should discuss their plans for pregnancy with their healthcare professionals. They should have a careful physical examination and laboratory studies to determine the activity of their lupus, as well as to check for the presence of antibodies (antiphospholipid antibodies and antibodies to Ro/SSA and La/SSB). In some cases, mothers with antiphospholipid antibodies will be placed on low-dose aspirin. If these mothers have had evidence of a previous blood clot, they may be treated with additional blood thinners along with aspirin during the pregnancy. These treatments have been shown to increase the chances of having a good pregnancy outcome.

Women with lupus should be monitored closely throughout the pregnancy by an obstetrician knowledgeable in high-risk pregnancies and a rheumatologist familiar with managing lupus. This team approach provides the best opportunity for mothers with lupus to have healthy full term babies.

8

Living and coping with lupus: tips for patients, family, and friends

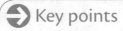 Key points

- Coping with lupus is not easy – it has many psychological, as well as physical, consequences.

- Patients need to understand as much about lupus as possible, in order to start trying to come to terms with it.

- For family, friends, and physicians, as well as the patient, education, education, education is the key to optimizing treatment.

There are many challenges faced by patients with lupus that often go beyond the physical limitations of the disease. Not only do patients have to deal with how they feel about their own illness but how other people respond to them. Emotional turmoil can begin with the onset of symptoms and before the diagnosis of lupus, and remain throughout the course of the disease. These relentless challenges can lead to fear, anxiety, and depression. This chapter will discuss the challenges of lupus and provide tips on how to cope with lupus, and how family and friends can help.

Patient's perspective

A very successful professor at a prestigious university told the story of how she kept her diagnosis of lupus a secret for years. She was fearful that her friends and colleagues would view her differently and that she would not be given the same opportunities for promotion and advancement if she were labelled with a chronic illness. It was only after she became highly successful in her profession that she stepped forward as a national lupus spokesperson. This is one example of how lupus patients fear 'social acceptability'. They are concerned about how society will view them and whether they will be accepted or rejected. Although this is not unique to lupus, and is seen in other chronic illnesses, there are certain features of lupus that make it particularly problematic.

First, lupus tends to target young women who are in the prime of their lives. They are often students, young mothers, or professionals who are climbing the ladder of success. People don't expect a young person to be sick and often have little tolerance for any sign of weakness.

Many lupus patients look well. They have no obvious physical signs of illness, even though they may be suffering considerably inside.

 Patient's perspective

During a recent programme at our university, an attractive woman with lupus explained to a group of young adults that she was undergoing chemotherapy for her kidney disease and suffered from arthritis and seizures. They were in disbelief. How can someone who looks so good be going through such hardship? Lupus patients often receive little empathy when they're feeling poorly. Many people around them are sceptical of the fatigue and may view them as lazy.

Unlike cancer, most people know very little about lupus and are not in a position to provide understanding or support.

Patient's perspective

One patient recently described how difficult it was for her when she was undergoing chemotherapy for her lupus. She was losing her hair, she was exhausted most days, and she was very frightened about her future. At the same time, her next door neighbour was receiving chemotherapy for breast cancer. Several of the women on her street ask her if she would like to join the group in planning meals for their friend with breast cancer. They discussed openly how devastated they were that their neighbour and friend had cancer. They felt compelled to help her. Of course she would join in and help with meals, but what about her own plight? Why did having lupus not generate the same emotion and concern in her neighbours and friends? Did they realize that there was a good chance that their friend with breast cancer would be cured and that lupus had no cure? Did they appreciate that lupus can be fatal? Ignorance and misconceptions about lupus can be trying for those afflicted with the disease.

Because lupus can be difficult to diagnose, many patients endure years of uncertainty and fear prior to the proper diagnosis being made.

 Patient's perspective

One patient described the years of her illness before being diagnosed as frightening. After the diagnosis she was still fearful at times, but she felt comfort in knowing why she was feeling ill and she gradually learned to deal with her lupus.

The fear of the unknown seems to be worse than knowing that you have lupus, although patients deal with some level of fear everyday. They fear the unpredictable flares of their disease, which make it difficult to make plans in advance. They fear maintaining employment, having children, and caring for their children. They also fear the financial consequences of a chronic illness like lupus. Many patients express concern about fulfilling roles as mother, father, worker, and lover. They don't want to lose their independence and they may feel guilty about the effects that their chronic illness has on loved ones and friends.

This rollercoaster of emotions can often lead to a clinical depression. Depression is a common problem in people with lupus. The causes for depression can be multifactorial, including:

- the stress of dealing with a chronic illness;

- the uncertainty and unpredictable nature of the disease;

- the sacrifices and limitations due to pain and fatigue;

- the strain on relationships with family and friends.

It is also important to point out that many of the medications used to treat lupus can also lead to depression, such as corticosteroids. Even manifestations of lupus may contribute to depression. Cognitive difficulties, memory loss, changes in personal appearance due to scarring skin rashes, hair loss or weight gain can add to the emotional distress. Unfortunately, depression often goes unrecognized in patients, since many of the symptoms of depression can be similar to the underlying disease. Some patients may deny that they are feeling unhappy or depressed, or they may feel uncomfortable discussing it with their physician. A good doctor–patient relationship can help patients open up and share their feelings, so that appropriate treatment can be started.

Here are few tips for living well with lupus:

- Learn as much as you possibly can about the disease – the unknown is always worse.

- Adopt a positive attitude and don't be hard on yourself. It is okay to take care of your needs and to adjust your daily schedule to meet them. It is also okay to take short naps when you need to refresh. If your job allows it, you can close your office door and put your head down on your desk for few minutes – you may need to keep a small alarm clock nearby. If appropriate, you may be able to adjust your work schedule to accommodate a short afternoon siesta or a later start in the morning.

- Don't be afraid to set goals for yourself and don't be too rigid. It is okay to make last-minute changes or to cancel plans. And remember – you don't have to keep apologizing!

◆ Learn how to deal with stressful situations – maybe by taking walks, practising yoga, meditation, biofeedback, or relaxing alone or with friends.

◆ Be sure to get enough rest, eat a well-balanced diet, and participate in a custom-designed exercise programme that is not too strenuous for you. And don't try to complete large tasks all at one time, tackle them one step at a time. This is a good rule for all of us!

◆ Most importantly, don't be afraid to seek help from a professional with any problems with anxiety, stress, fear, or depression that you feel you are unable to manage on your own. There is plenty of help out there.

How can family and friends help?

Keep in mind that your family and friends may be overwhelmed and just as frightened as you with your diagnosis, and they may have a difficult time understanding and adapting to inevitable changes. They may feel helpless and afraid. There may be frustration, since the traditional roles and responsibilities, particularly within families, may change when a member of the family has a chronic illness.

Here are a few tips for helping friends and family live well with lupus:

◆ Educate family members and friends about the disease. It is extremely helpful if they accompany you to your doctors' appointments, so that they can hear what your doctor says and they can ask questions. If necessary, talk to your doctor ahead of time and explain that you need help in conveying certain issues about lupus to your loved ones. This is an ideal time for your doctor to explain the unpredictable nature of the disease and the profound fatigue that is common in lupus. They should hear your doctor say that you are not 'faking' your fatigue, and that you really do need to rest frequently. If your family can appreciate how important their love and support are in managing lupus and preventing the stress that can flare disease, they have an easier time adjusting to changes in their routine. Be sure that your family and friends understand the side-effects of the medications that you are taking, so that they can be aware of, and recognize, problems that may arise. Some medications may also affect your emotional state and this may help them understand if your behaviour changes radically.

◆ It is important that everyone speak openly and honestly with each other. These conversations should be as positive as possible, without placing blame and avoiding anger. You are certainly not to blame for your lupus. It is not uncommon for your family, especially children, to look to you for strength. If they see that you are giving up, they may become frightened or angry. This may cause them to escape or retreat and leave you feeling alone. Keeping a positive attitude helps everyone, even when you are having your own doubts.

◆ Keep in mind that it takes time for family and friends to adapt to the physical, emotional and lifestyle changes that are happening to a loved one.

◆ Remember that there is group and family counselling available for families who are struggling.

9

The factors that conspire to cause lupus

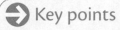

> ## Key points
>
> ◆ A combination of factors 'conspire' to cause lupus.
>
> ◆ These factors include genetic, hormonal, and environmental elements.
>
> ◆ The precise way in which these factors 'conspire' are not fully established.

Introduction

> ## Fact
>
> Patients frequently ask the 'why me' question – with its subtext 'and why not my relative or friend!?'
>
> While an entirely reasonable question, and in spite of great increases in our knowledge, it cannot be fully answered. However, it is clear that a number of factors conspire to cause lupus and we will consider them in this chapter.

As a simple analogy to help understand the problem, imagine a pack of cards. The name of the game is 'health'.

The 'health' game

The cards are not marked with the conventional titles, e.g. ace of spades, 2 of diamonds, 3 of clubs, etc., but rather with titles such as female sex, male sex, age 10–20, age 50–60, genetic factor X or Y, exposure to high-fat diet, exposure to low-fat diet, stress and so on.

The cards are shuffled and if the hand that you are dealt consists of something like:

- female sex card;

- aged 15–40 card;

- genetic ability to make anti-dsDNA antibodies;

- exposure to Epstein–Barr virus;

- high, saturated-fat diet;

- genetic factor HLA-B8;

- genetic factor HLA-DR3;

then you have just been dealt a lupus hand! (see Fig. 9.1).

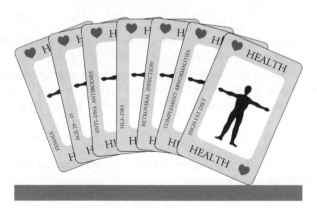

Figure 9.1 Factors causing lupus – the card game for adults.

It should thus be evident that lupus is not the consequence of a single fault or problem within the body, but rather the consequence of the interaction of a large number of factors that conspire to bring about the disease. The analogy also reminds us that a deck of cards can easily be re-shuffled and factors that conspire to cause lupus are rather similar to those cause other autoimmune diseases. Thus it is notable that 30% of patients with lupus do develop one or more additional autoimmune diseases, such as Sjögren's syndrome, myositis, and antiphospholipid antibody syndrome.

The most important cards or factors are as follows:

- sex hormones;

- genetics;

- trigger factors;

- diet;

- stress.

Sex hormones

 Fact

It is very striking that females are approximately 10 times more likely to get lupus than males, between the ages of 15 and 50. Before 15 and after 50 the female-to-male ratio falls to around 3 or 4 to 1. These simple facts carry the strong implication that female sex hormones are providing a critical 'environment' for the development of lupus.

It has been established that there are close links between the endocrine (hormone) and the immune system. For example, female sex hormones have the ability to stimulate the helper T lymphocytes, so-called because they help B lymphocytes to produce antibodies. In contrast, male sex hormones encourage suppressor T lymphocytes, which tend to block the production of antibodies.

Based on the presumption that female sex hormones do provide one of the important factors in the 'lupus conspiracy', attempts have been made, to change the hormonal environment in patients with lupus in the hope of treating the disease. However, there are almost certainly subtleties at play here, which might explain why our attempts to date have achieved a rather modest degree of success.

Genetics

Very simple observations with identical and non-identical twins point to the importance of genetic factors. Consider a lupus patient who we will call Mary. When Mary's twin sister comes to us and asks what is her chance of getting lupus, if the twins are identical, the chance is 25%, but if they are not identical, it is approximately 2–3%. This tells us two things:

1. Genes are important because the difference between the identical twins, i.e. twins having essentially the same genes, is about nine times higher than those twins who are not identical, i.e. they have different sets of genes.

2. Importantly, this information also implies that genes alone are not sufficient to cause the disease, because if they were, the chances of Mary's identical twin sister developing lupus would be close to 100%, when in fact the real figure is only a quarter of that.

Other family studies have indicated the importance of genetic predisposition. Thus, for example, among the first 400 lupus patients followed up at University College Hospital in London, 15 are known to have sisters with lupus and four of these patients had mothers or daughters with the disease.

A major attempt is being made by groups in North America and in Europe, using the results of the human-genome scan, to identify the particular genes that are critical to the development of the disease. It seems likely that over a dozen such genes will be involved and these are likely to include:

◆ genes that ensure cells die at an appropriate time (the apoptosis genes);

◆ genes that regulate small marker proteins on the surface of cells known as the major histocompatibility complex (MHC) genes; and

◆ genes that regulate key inflammatory molecules, the cytokines.

Within the next 10 years we will probably have a very accurate idea of exactly which genes are critical for the development of lupus.

Among these relevant genes, we are also likely to find those that regulate the production of harmful autoantibodies, i.e. antibodies that bind to the body's own tissues.

 Fact

Antibodies, also known as immunoglobulins, are divided into five families or classes:

- IgG
- IgM
- IgA
- IgD
- IgE.

Curiously individuals who have an inherited inability to produce the IgA class are more likely to develop autoimmune diseases, including lupus, although the reason for this is uncertain.

Those antibodies that bind to material found in the cell nucleus, especially the nucleosome and dsDNA alone, are already strongly suspected of being deeply involved in the development of SLE.

 Fact

The nucleosome consists of double-stranded (ds) DNA and histones, the protein that DNA naturally wraps around.

These antibodies have been identified in the kidney tissues both of mice, which get a form of lupus, and lupus patients. While that places them at the 'scene of the crime', it does not prove that they 'pulled the trigger'. However, evidence has been gathered from a variety of experiments that does suggest that these antibodies do carry the 'smoking gun'. The genetics of antibody production are complicated and will not be described here. Suffice it to say that, although healthy individuals may produce some autoantibodies, they are kept at a low level and are of the IgM type. In contrast, the ability to produce antibodies of the IgG class is more concerning, since these are the antibodies are generally associated with pathological effects. Thus, those individuals whose genes dictate that they are better able to produce IgG antibodies to self-antigens, are also probably more likely to develop lupus.

It is however, of great interest that the antibodies that we associate with lupus (such as anti-dsDNA, anti-Ro, anti-Sm, for example) have been shown (by John Harley and colleagues in Oklahoma) to be detectable in the blood of lupus patients for several years prior to the development of clinical features of lupus. This is further proof that no single factor will cause the disease. Further evidence is provided by the fact that some malignant tumours of plasma cells (those cells that actually make antibodies) known as myelomas, produce large quantities of what are actually autoantibodies without the patient developing the disease that is often associated with that antibody. Thus, patients with myeloma may have 20 g/l (a large amount!) of rheumatoid factor without developing rheumatoid arthritis and equally large amounts of IgG anti-dsDNA antibodies without getting lupus.

Trigger factors

The best known trigger factor for lupus is exposure to ultraviolet radiation (sunlight). As mentioned in Chapter 1, this factor was first recognized in 1879 by an English physician called Hutchinson. What was not known until recently was why this phenomenon occurred. We now understand that ultraviolet radiation has the ability to increase the rate at which cells die, by a complicated process known as apoptosis. One consequence of apoptosis is a kind of turning inside-out of the cell, so that the nuclear material usually found deep within the cell becomes exposed on the surface. However, cells that have died as a consequence of apoptosis are usually recognized and removed very swiftly by macrophage cells (part of the white cell family). Thus, the nuclear-protein fragments appear on the cell surface for very short periods of time and generally excite no 'interest' from other cells of the immune system. It is now recognized that the normal mechanisms for getting rid of dead and dying cells are inefficient in patients with lupus. Fragments of the nucleus, including DNA, are picked up by other immune system cells and this leads, through a somewhat complicated pathway, to the production of antibodies against these nuclear fragments, including anti-DNA antibodies. By simple analogy, think of the situation in which garbage (rubbish) collectors go out on strike and fail to pick up the weekly garbage. In a week or two the garbage bins begin to overflow and this seems to be what is happening in patients who develop lupus.

Whatever the precise mechanism for autoantibody production, it is self-evident that the avoidance of excessive amounts of sun exposure does play an important (non-pharmacological) part in the treatment of lupus (as described in Chapter 6).

Other factors that may trigger lupus include certain drugs and quite possibly some viral infections. Several sulphur-based drugs and some older anti-hypertensive drugs (e.g. hydralazine), and drugs used in the treatment of tuber-culosis (e.g. isoniazid) have been described, almost certainly, in genetically susceptible individuals, to cause a lupus-like disease. Patients with drug-induced lupus tend to get the skin and joint manifestations of the disease but, more rarely, if at all, the kidney and central nervous system manifestations.

Investigators in the United States have provided evidence that the Epstein–Barr virus (which is responsible for infectious mononucleosis/glandular fever) could be an important trigger, especially in younger patients with lupus. Since some lupus patients do give a clear-cut history that their disease seems to have developed, or may worsen, following a flu-like illness, it is also possible that other viruses could act as a trigger, quite possibly through the mechanism of increasing the rate of cell death (apoptosis). However, trying to determine which among the hundreds, if not thousands, of known viruses might be responsible, does equate to finding needles in hay stacks!

Diet

Many patients are intrigued to know whether diet could be responsible for their lupus. As indicated from the card-game analogy earlier this is clearly not the whole story but there are some data to suggest that diet may be contributory. Over 20 years ago, John Morrow and Jay Levy in San Francisco took mice, genetically programmed to develop a form of lupus, and did nothing except to alter the content of the diet that they were fed. By reducing the saturated-fat content of the diet, they showed that these mice lived a little longer, had less kidney disease, and lower levels of antibodies to DNA. By analogy, a study undertaken at University College London showed a statistically significant benefit for patients taking a combination of a low-fat diet (the saturated-fat content of the diet was reduced from over 35% to less than 25%), together with fish oils (which contain relatively large amounts of omega-3 fatty acids).

Some patients are convinced that reducing gluten in their diet may be helpful. Other patients become convinced that particular types of foods may be triggering their disease but the evidence for this is not very compelling.

Stress

Another question that is commonly asked of physicians looking after patients with lupus is whether stress might be responsible for the disease or involved in disease flares. There is no 'stress-o-meter' that would reliably measure levels of stress in human beings and clearly what is stressful for one person is not stressful for another. Attempts have been made in patients with a variety of autoimmune diseases to determine whether these diseases were more likely to have begun after events such as moving house, examinations, divorce – all generally acknowledged to be stressful. Although no terribly clear-cut answers have been derived from this research, there remains a perception that, for some patients at least, stress may be one of the factors in the development of lupus. Much larger studies over longer periods of time are needed before the existence of this factor could be regarded as completely convincing.

10

The current outlook for lupus patients and why the future is getting brighter

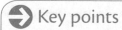 Key points

- We are living in an exciting era in which increased knowledge of the key molecules causing the features of lupus, together with new technologies, are leading to the introduction of a host of new therapies for SLE.

- There is genuine hope that these new approaches will provide effective and safe alternatives to steroids and the use of the older immunosuppressive drugs.

- Many of the new drugs are undergoing large-scale clinical trials.

Introduction

In the 1950s, lupus was widely regarded as a fatal disease. The chances that a patient diagnosed with lupus would live for 5 years were only 50% – the equivalent to many patients with different sorts of cancer. However, the prognosis for lupus patients is now much improved, so that an average survival after diagnosis of 15–20 years is the norm in around 80% of patients.

How was this improvement brought about?

Undoubtedly the introduction of corticosteroids and other drugs that suppress the immune system have made a big difference to patients with more severe lupus. Corticosteroids were introduced at the Mayo Clinic (for the treatment of rheumatoid arthritis initially) in the late 1940s but were being widely used for lupus patients by the mid to late 1950s. It took a while, however, before the serious side-effects (osteoporosis, increased risk of infection, diabetes, hypertension) on large doses of steroids, used for long periods of time, were widely recognized. Undoubtedly, the optimal dose of steroids is the lowest possible dose, for the shortest possible period of time. However, the potential life-saving capacity of corticosteroids for lupus patients with, say, low levels of platelets, low haemoglobin, and aggressive renal disease, should not be underestimated. The introduction of drugs like azathioprine and methotrexate and cyclophosphamide in the 1960s, cyclosporin in the 1980s and mycophenolate in the 1990s have all made a significant contribution to improve survival, notably in patients with renal lupus, which was the commonest cause of death in lupus patients in the 1950s.

By the mid-1970s, it had become evident that patients with lupus who did die could be divided into two groups:

(1) those dying in the early years of their disease were succumbing to very active lupus (though a contribution to the deaths of these patients from infection, brought about, at least in part, by the immunosuppressive drugs, should be recognized);

(2) deaths occurring in patients who had had the disease for much longer, over 15–20 years.

In the second group of patients, it became evident that atherosclerosis – a kind of furring up of the blood vessels, notably the arteries restricting blood flow to the heart muscle and other parts of the body – was making a major contribution to lupus deaths.

More accurate determination of lupus deaths due to heart attacks has shown that a highly significant increased risk is evident from the age of 35 upwards; indeed patients with lupus aged between 35 and 45 are 50 times more likely to develop a heart attack. As discussed in Chapter 3, the exact reason for this substantial increase remains uncertain. To reiterate what has been established, is that some conventional risk factors for heart attacks, such as heavy smoking, diabetes, a family history of heart attacks, and strokes, are not more common among patients with lupus compared with the normal population. The Systemic

Lupus International Collaborating Clinics (SLICC) group is undertaking a major international long-term follow-up study to try and seek answers to this important question.

The increased risk of heart attacks (and to a lesser extent strokes) has remained a considerable threat to patients with lupus over the past 30 years. Relatively few patients, however, die directly from kidney disease any more, and one recent study at University College Hospital London has reported that amongst those who do, poor adherence to treatment is a significant contributing factor. The problem of ensuring that patients take the medication prescribed is a particular problem amongst adolescents and those in their early twenties. It is very understandable that young women, in particular, do not easily accept some of the side-effects associated with corticosteroids, notably swelling of the face and weight gain. In addition, many women are naturally concerned about the threats to their ability to conceive and sustain pregnancies, which can be threatened by several of the standard immunosuppressive drugs, as well as activity of the disease itself. Nevertheless, these drugs have contributed enormously to the considerable increase in survival of patients with lupus.

A major aim of treatment is to seek a balance between effective disease control and drug side-effects. Patient education is an important part of this effort. Thus, as a matter of routine, the significant side-effects of powerful immuno-suppressive drugs need to be discussed with patients, the warning signs of possible problems emphasized, and patient information sheets provided, so the patients may go home and study them in more detail. However, patients also need to be aware of what might be called the 'Clouseau' effect.

The 'Clouseau' effect

Imagine that the famous detective has been chasing a villain around the streets of Paris. The villain runs into a small hotel. Clouseau follows him. Standing in the front hall of the hotel Clouseau cannot see the villain, but is convinced that he must have run through a narrow doorway off the hall. However, standing in the doorway is a fierce looking dog. 'Monsieur', says Clouseau to the owner of the hotel sitting behind the reception desk, 'does your dog bite?'

'No' is the reply.

'Eh bien' says Clouseau, who then runs to the doorway but is outraged when the dog takes a bite at his backside.

'Monsieur, I thought you said your dog does not bite!'

'Yes, inspector, but this is not my dog!'

In other words, just because a patient has started a new drug it does not mean that every thing that happens subsequently is the fault of the drug. As an example, a patient attending the lupus clinic at University College Hospital called to say that 2 days after starting azathioprine she had come out in a rash. On examination, however, the 'rash' was typical of insect bites and it transpired that the day after starting the drug the patient had gone camping for the night with her young daughter. The 'rash' faded in a few days and the drug was continued successfully.

The commonest cause of death in patients with lupus today are:

◆ infection;

◆ atherosclerosis/vascular disease;

◆ cancer.

Severely active disease on its own, notably kidney disease, now comes some way down the list. The risk of an infection relates in many cases to the prolonged use of drugs that suppress the immune system. Unfortunately, these drugs suppress in a very non-specific way and, although they can be very effective at persuading the immune system to stop attacking the body's own tissues, they do increase the likelihood of infection from a wide variety of viruses and bacteria, which may on occasion prove fatal.

The links between lupus and cancer are being re-assessed. The SLICC group has recently reviewed 10 000 patients under long term follow-up with lupus looking in great detail for cases of cancer and comparing the rates of the various types of cancer in patients with lupus and matched healthy controls. While, overall, there was very little difference in the cancer risk between the lupus patients and the matched healthy controls, there was a small increase in a cancer called non-Hodgkin's lymphoma and, to a lesser extent, with lung cancer. Intriguingly, the patients who developed non-Hodgkin's lymphoma tended to do so within the first year or two of their lupus diagnosis. The study did not find a major increase in patients with lupus who had been treated with immunosuppressive drugs for a number of years (a concern that had been expressed by some prior to this study), although even longer term studies will be needed to confirm these data.

Why the future looks brighter

The keys to our optimism about the future include:

◆ a 'happy coalition' of improved understanding of the causes of lupus plus;

◆ a greater willingness on the part of major pharmaceutical companies to get involved in developing new therapies; and

◆ the willingness of the lupus research community to work together to develop new, validated, and reliable 'tools' to assess patients with lupus.

The remarkable advances in our understanding of the causes of diseases, including lupus, has enabled the identification of key molecules that are thought to play a leading role in its development. An analogy can be made with patients who have rheumatoid arthritis, in whom it has been shown that a small molecule called TNF-α (a member of the cytokine protein family) is essential in the development of the inflamed joints. Three widely used drugs that block the effects of TNF-α have been developed and, in each case, around 70% of patients who have failed to respond adequately to older, more conventional drugs (such as methotrexate and salazopyrine) are significantly improved by them.

Several molecules have been identified that are now widely believed to be essential in the development of SLE. The immunological pathway and places where new drugs, mostly biological agents, are directed is shown in Fig. 10.1. Biological agents (monoclonal antibodies) have been produced that block the effects of these molecules; these have been given to a small number of lupus patients with some apparent success. The hope is that these biological agents, by targeting individual small molecules, might prove analogous to the TNF-α blockers in rheumatoid arthritis and be able to provide benefits equal to those of steroids and immunosuppressive drugs but without the major side-effects that these more conventional drugs are known to cause. It will, sadly, be some years before we can be certain about this, however.

As mentioned briefly in Chapter 5, prominent among these new approaches is a biological agent known as rituximab (which binds and blocks a molecule known as CD20 present on most B lymphocytes), originally developed for the treatment of non-Hodgkin's lymphoma, which has been combined (in many although not all patients) with cyclophosphamide and steroids. Several thousand patients around the world in different centres have shown a significant beneficial response with very few side-effects. The results of a double-blind, control trial, currently ongoing in North America, are awaited with great interest.

Lupus · the**facts**

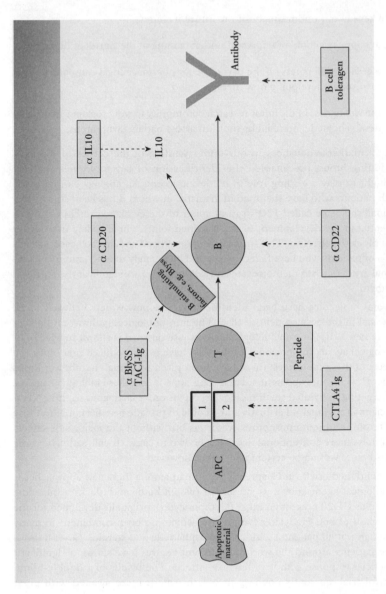

Figure 10.1 Places where intervention is being tried in the immunological pathway leading to lupus.

In addition to the above approaches, a variety of others, including biological agents that block molecules which activate B lymphocytes (e.g. Belimumab) and others that interfere with the link between T-lymphocyte cells and those that can present fragments of protein or other antigens (antigen presenting cells) (abatacept), have also been tried out in patients with lupus. Other new drugs include attempts to block the effects of anti-dsDNA antibodies (e.g. abatemis sodium and teraparatide).

It will be evident from the above that we are moving into the age of the biological therapy in which, having identified key molecules likely to be involved in the development of different diseases, biological agents can be created that, in effect, block these molecules and should therefore stand a chance of success-fully treating the particular disease. The recent experience at Northwick Park Hospital in London confirms (a most unfortunate episode in which an anti-body to a protein marker, known as CD28, on a T lymphocyte caused very severe side-effects in healthy controls) that we will face some challenging problems to improve still further the outlook for patients with lupus. However, we are confident that in 5 years time possibly, 10 years time probably, and 15 years time definitely, the treatment of patients with lupus will have changed quite radically, with a much more widespread and earlier use of biological agents.

We surmise that the increased willingness of the drug companies to get involved in lupus research is partly because they recognize that there are suffi-cient numbers of patients with the disease to make it worth their while. In addition, some potentially useful drugs (such as rituximab) had already been produced for other reasons, which saves vast amounts of money in drug-development costs. Similarly, it is also quite possible that drugs developed ostensibly for treating patients with lupus, might also be useful in the treat-ment of other autoimmune diseases.

Well before it became apparent that new biological agents were likely to become available for the treatment of patients with lupus, research groups around the world had begun to collaborate. Thus the SLICC group, in partic-ular, formed in 1991, has worked tirelessly to develop, compare, and recom-mend the type of assessment tools that can be used in long-term observational studies of lupus patients and in trials of new therapies. It is now generally accepted that to capture the totality of the effect of a disease like lupus on a patient, we need an activity index, a damage index, and a patient-perception index. By activity we mean, principally, clinical features due to on-going inflammation. By damage we refer to permanent change that has developed since the diagnosis of the disease was made (this could have a variety of causes including previous disease activity, drug effects, or other concomitant disorders).

Capturing the patients' view of their disease is also vital, as it is likely to differ from that of their physician! Virtually all of the on-going trials of new therapies in lupus are using the British Isles Lupus Assessment (BILA) activity index (this index assesses lupus activity within eight organs or systems) often accompanied by a global score measure known as SLEDAI (Systemic Lupus Erythematosus Disease Activity Index); the SLICC/ACR damage index, and a patient healthcare assessment measure known as the SF-36. Again we surmise that this generally uniform approach to disease assessment is attractive to the pharmaceutical companies, who do not have to go out and develop new tools.

11

Lupus myths and fables

As physicians who have spent many years working in lupus clinics we have become aware of many 'myths and fables' about the disease itself, its outlook and its treatment. We'd like to set the record straight as far as possible. We don't have all the answers and, tragically for some, lupus is a fatal disease or one that causes great hardship. Our responses to concerns that have been expressed to us are based as far as possible on established facts; though the odd prejudice may slip in!

❌ Common myths about lupus

❌ **Myth:** Lupus? – It's a fatal disease.

❗ **Fact:** In the 1950s the 5-year survival for patients with lupus was 50%, i.e. 1 patient in 2 would die within 5 years. It is now around 85% 15-year survival. Many patients with lupus live to a 'ripe old age'. However, about 15% of the patients at UCH in London followed for up to 25 years, have died, with an average age of 51 years, ranging from 16 to 87. A relatively small number of lupus patients thus continue to die far too young.

❌ **Myth:** Lupus destroys your kidneys.

❗ **Fact:** Out of 401 patients with lupus looked after for up to 25 years at the Middlesex/UCH in London, only 21 went into kidney failure (requiring dialysis and in some cases transplantation). Of these 21, at least half were poorly adherent to treatment. In other words patients, especially if diagnosed early, who maintain their treatment (especially if they control their blood pressure) are extremely unlikely to destroy their kidneys.

❌ **Myth:** Having lupus means you can never go out in sunlight.

❗ **Fact:** It's true that patients with lupus (notably those with white/ light brown skin) must be careful. Many patients are photosensitive. However, we do not advocate that lupus patients confine their holidays to 2 weeks in Greenland during December! Any patients, especially those with a history of a rash, should take sensible precautions. Avoid the hottest, sunniest resorts in the middle of summer; wear wide-brimmed hats to shield the face and use lots of sun screens (factor 25 or greater). Remember that driving in a car with your arm on an open window-ledge can also cause problems.

❌ **Myth:** Lupus goes after 50.

❗ **Fact:** It's true that for many patients with SLE the onset of the meno-pause signals (almost certainly by virtue of the lowered oestrogen levels) a distinct improvement in their symptoms. However, this is not true for all patients and, paradoxically, around 5% of patients with SLE are diagnosed over the age of 50.

❌ **Myth:** Its dangerous for a lupus patient to take oestrogen to stop the symptoms of the menopause.

❗ **Fact:** There are some descriptions of patients with lupus taking post-menopausal hormones and developing flares of their disease. However, it is now evident that this is *not* the case for most patients. Probably 6 of 7 patients who 'enter' the menopause can take oestro-gen without causing their lupus to flare, although caution *is* needed for these patients suspected of having an increased risk of thrombosis.

❌ **Myth:** I've got lupus and I've been told not to have children.

❗ **Fact:** Most lupus patients have normal fertility. In the absence of active kidney disease there is no reason not to consider starting a family with the following caveats:

◆ If you are on cyclophosphamide, methotrexate, and probably myco-phenolate, you will need to stop medication for 3 months before trying to get pregnant.

◆ You should ensure careful monitoring during pregnancy. Some, but not all, reports suggest that there may be an increased flare rate during pregnancy.

◆ If you have anticardiolipin (or other antiphospholipid) antibodies there is an increased risk of losing your baby. This problem can be prevented using a combination of aspirin and heparin but your disease will need to be managed carefully by your obstetrician and rheumatologist.

◆ If you have anti-Ro or anti-La antibodies there is a 1:20 chance that your body will have the 'neonatal lupus syndrome', which leads to a rash (which usually goes within 2-3 weeks) and 'heart block' (a condition in which the heart beats irregularly) and may well require a pace-maker.

Appendix
World lupus group organizations

AUSTRALIA

The Lupus Association of NSW Inc.
P.O. Box 89
North Ryde NSW 1670
Australia
Tel: +612 9878 6055
Fax: +612 9878 6049
info@lupusnsw.org.au
sjogrens@lupusnsw.org.au
http://www.lupusnsw.org.au

Lupus Australia Foundation Inc
2nd Floor, Rosee House
247 Flinders Lane
Melbourne 3001
Australia
Tel: +613 9560 5348
Fax: +613 9663 4210
vla@lupusvic.org
http://www.lupusvic.org.au

WESTERN AUSTRALIA

Lupus Group of Western Australia Inc.
Royal Perth Hospital
C/- P.O. Box X2213
Perth, W.A. 6847
Australia

Fax: +618-9224-3144
lupus@wanet.com.au
http://www.lupuswa.com.au

Lupus Association of Tasmania
P.O. Box 639
Launceston, Tasmania 7250
Australia
Tel: +613-6331-9940
lupustas@bigpond.net.au
http://www.users.bigpond.net.au/
lupustas

CANADA

Lupus Canada
590 Alden Road Suite 211
Markham
Ontario
L3R 8N2
Toll Free (in Canada):
1-800-661-1468
Tel: +1905-513-0004
Fax: +1905-513-9516
lupuscanada@beilnet.ca
http://www.lupuscanada.org

MAURITIUS
Lupus Alert
E111 Clos Verger
Rose Hill
Rep of Mauritius
Tel: +230 464 8276
lupusalert@hotmail.com

NEW ZEALAND
**Lupus Association of
New Zealand**
C/- Arthritis & Rheumatism
Foundation of New Zealand Inc.
P.O. Box 10-020
Wellington
New Zealand

Lupus Care and Support Inc.
P.O. Box 72578
Papakura, Auckland
New Zealand
http://www.lupus.org.nz

UNITED STATES OF AMERICA
Alliance for Lupus Research
28 West 44th Street, Suite 501,
New York, NY 10036
Tel: +1 212 218 2840
info@lupusresearch.org
http://www.lupusresearch.org

Lupus Alliance of America
Long Island/Queens Affiliate
2255 Centre Avenue,
Bell more, New York 11710
Tel: +1516-783-3370 or 1800-850-
9000 or +1516-826-2058
info@lupusli.org
http://www.lupusliqueens.org

**Lupus Foundation of America
Inc.**
National Office,
2000 L Street, N.W., Suite 710
Washington, DC 20036
Tel: +1202-349-1155
Fax: +1202-349-1156
info@lupus.org
http://www.lupus.org

Lupus Research Institute
330 Seventh Avenue, Suite 1701
New York, NY 10001
Tel: +1 212 812 9881
Fax: +1 212 545 1843
Lupus@LupusNY.org
http://www.lupusresearchinstitute.org

ELEF MEMBER COUNTRIES
(European Lupus Erythematosus
Federation)

BELGIUM (FLEMISH LANG)
**League for Chronic
Inflammatory Connective Tissue
Diseases**
CiB-Liga vzw
Lindenlaan 15
B-3680 Maaseik
Belgium
Tel./Fax: +32-89-50-3108
secretariat@cibliga.be
http://www.cibliga.be

BELGIUM (FRENCH LANG)

**Lupus Erythematosus
Association**
Avenue des Jardins 62 bte. 19
B 1030 Brussels
Belgium
Tel: +32-2-726 51 41
http://www.lupus-belgium.org

CYPRUS

**Cyprus League Against
Rheumatism**
P.O. Box 24966
Nicosia 1306
Cyprus
cyplar@cytanet.com.cy
http://www.rheumatism.org.cy

DENMARK

**SLE-Group, The Danish
Rheumatism Association**
Gentoftegade 118
DK-2820 Gentofte
Denmark
Tel: +45-39-77 80 00
http://www.gigtforeningen.dk

FINLAND

Finnish SLE-Group co.
The Finnish Rheumatism
Association
C/- The Finnish Rheumatism
Association
Iso Roobertinkatu 20 – 22A
FIN-00120 Helsinki
Finland
Tel: +358-9 4761 55
Fax: +358-9 642 286
info@reumaliitto.fi
http://www.reumaliitto.fi

FRENCH

**The French Association of
Lupus sufferers and
autoimmune diseases**
34, rue Principale Lemestroff
F-57970 Oudrenne
France
Tel: +33-82-55 0923
lupusplus@gmail.com

LUPUS France
Rue de Rocroy 7
F-75010 Paris
France
Tel/ Fax: +33-1-45 26 33 27
presidente@lupusfrance.fr
http://www.lupusfrance.fr

GERMANY

**Lupus Erythematosus Self help
Association**
Doeppersberg 20
42103 Wuppertal
Germany
Tel: +49-202-496 87 97
Fax: +49-202-496 87 98
lupus@rheumanet.org or
leshg@lupus-rheumanet.org
http://www.lupus.rheumanet.org

ICELAND

The Lupus Group of the Icelandic League against Rheumatism
The Icelandic League against Rheumatism
Armuli 5
IS-108 Reykjavik
Iceland
Tel: +-354-530-36 00
Fax: +354-553-07 65
http://www.gigt.is

IRELAND

Irish Lupus Support Group Limited
Carmichael Centre
North Brunswick Street
Dublin 7
Ireland
Tel: +353-1-872 45 18
Fax: +353-1-873 57 37
irishupus@iol.ie
http://www.lupus.ie

ISRAEL

Israeli Lupus Association (ILA)
P.O.Box 14103
Tel Aviv 61141
Israel
Tel: +972-3-677-33 46
Fax: +972-3-635-44 64
lupus@drc.co.il
http://www.lupus.org.il

ITALY

Italian SLE Group
Via Arbotori, 14
I 29100 Piacenza
Italy
Tel: +39-0523-75 36 43
Fax: +39-0523-75 36 43
info@lupus-italy.org
http://www.lupus-italy.org/

MALTA

Lupus Support Group Malta
St Paul's Garden
IX-Xwieki
L/o Gharghur, NXR 09
Malta, GC
Tel: +356-21 370 234
Fax: +356-21 377 402
elizian@vol.net.mt

THE NETHERLANDS

National Society LE Patients
Bisonspoor 3004
NL-3605 LV Maarssen
The Netherlands
Tel: +31-346-55 24 01
Fax: +31-346-56 92 73
info@nvle.org
http://www.nvle.org

NORWAY

Lupus Foundation within NRF
Bekkeveien 11
N-0667 Oslo
Norway
Tel: +47-22-75 81 56
flavoll@online.no

PORTUGAL

Association of Patients with SLE
Avenida Defensores de Chaves
No. 27 4. Dto
P-1000-110 Lisboa
Portugal
Tel: +351-21-330 26 40
Fax: +351-21-314 62 16
associacao.lupus@clix.pt
http://www.lupus.saudeglobal.com

SPAIN

Spanish Lupus Association
C/- Lagunillas, 25
Locales 3 y 4
E-29012 Málaga
Spain
Tel/Fax: +34-952-25 08 26
felupus@felupus.org
http://www.felupus.org

SWEDEN

The SLE-Sjögren-group
Retimatikerförbundet
Box 128 51
119 98 Stockholm
Sweden
Tel: +46-8505 805 12
kerstin.kailander@
reumatikerforbundet.org
http://www.reumatikerforbundet.org

SWITZERLAND

Swiss Lupus Erythematosus Association
Niesenstrasse 9
CH-3062 Worb
Switzerland
Tel: +41-31-839 69 76
me.rosch@gmx.ch
http://www.slev.ch

UNITED KINGDOM

Lupus UK
St. James House
27–43, Eastern Road
Romford/Essex
RMI 3NH
United Kingdom
Tel: +44-1708-73-12-51
Fax: +44-1708-73-12-52
chris@lupusuk.org.uk
http://www.lupusuk.org.uk

Index